THE
GOD
THAT
WE'VE
CREATED

To Barbara —

" For this cause have you come "

Michael O'Donnell

THE
GOD
THAT
WE'VE
CREATED

അ

The Basic Cause
of all
DISEASE

by Michele Longo O'Donnell

LA VIDA PRESS
SAN ANTONIO

Library of Congress Card Number:
2005920245

ISBN 0-9676861-5-6 hardcover
ISBN 0-9676861-4-8 softcover

Published in 2005 by
La Vida Press
410 West Craig Place
San Antonio, Texas 78212
888-493-8660

Cover design and illustration by Travis Ward

Printed in USA

*This is dedicated to all the Peggys and Rays
of the world, who need to hear the truth to live.
May this reach their hearts.*

T HE STATELY TREE SEEN ON THE COVER *is a Cedar of Lebanon. Rich with symbolism, poets and writers alike liken it to the true nature of man as seen from the eyes of his Creator.*

When King Solomon built Israel's first Temple in the 10th century B.C., he wanted it to reflect God's majesty, so he used the finest materials available: gold, silver and cedar wood from Lebanon.

Throughout the Bible man is referred to as a Cedar of Lebanon. Symbolic of strength and beauty, it reminds man of his inherent nature, brought forth in the very image and likeness of his Creator.

The Cedar of Lebanon grows and flourishes, springing out from the dry, desert sands. This is our promise that no matter how forbearing and bleak may be the circumstances of our lives, we too can expect to burst forth, reaching for the sunlight of Life. This also demonstrates that our situations are not to govern our experiences, but our lives are to be an unbroken expression of the Life of God which is our life and our breath. The desert sand cannot give life, but the Spirit of Life within us will, eternally.

The word Lebanon literally means purification and white. The Cedar speaks to man of his strength, grandeur and ability to survive and flourish wherever planted. The cedar is a tree not subject to decay, also repelling insects and worms. Therefore we read in the Song of Solomon 1:17, to make the "beams of our house cedar" is to preserve the mind, the body and the soul of man from corruption.

Just like the Cedar of Lebanon, all creation speaks to man of his true nature and identity. The knowledge of this will preserve man from evil. But in the absence of this understanding, "man will eat the very sand."

TABLE OF CONTENTS

SECTION 2

SECTION 3

Section 5

Section 6

ACKNOWLEDGEMENTS

It takes a community effort to write a book. Everyone within the radius of my life ends up assisting. The focus which is required is rather intense causing the needs of the immediate family to barely get scratched. Consequently everyone ends up carrying my load as well as their own and there doesn't seem to be any way around that.

The person that I want to thank first is my husband, George. He picked up the slack and never missed a beat. He remained patient and totally supportive, giving me the space I needed to finish the work. I never had to worry about the house falling down around me. He did a wonderful job and I thank him from the depths of my heart.

At the clinic I think they have forgotten what I look like. I showed up so infrequently during this time and although I met and interview each one, the faces and names became a blur, as did the rest of my life. I thank God every day for Melissa Raymond, who long ago took the reins for me and has done a job that no one on this earth could match.

She has become the heart and the soul of the work down there. She and her crew deserve an award for their dedication to the place, to the patients and to the vision given to me so many years ago.

My assistant, Kay Wynne is another indispensable soul, without whose devotion to me I could have never done this. She managed my books, my tapes, my traveling schedule, airline tickets and hotel rooms. She handled my radio shows, TV shows and everything else that we are involved with. Everyone should have a Kay and I thank God that I do!

It was important to me that the writings be reviewed by someone who understood the message and understood my heart's desire to share the truths. Once again my faithful friend, Melissa, jumped in as she always does and spent the long days and nights editing for me. Another person that I must mention, who certainly took my English grammar to task is my friend and pastor, Rev. Linda Marcella Whitsett.

Last, I want to mention my good friend, Debbie McClain, who came up with the idea for the cover. It was truly an inspiration, as it encompassed exactly the message of the book.

Many people who have gone before me have influenced my thinking and enabled me to build upon their understandings. This is a new revelation to the inhabitance of the earth and like any new thought we receive it line upon line and precept upon precept as we are able to comprehend it. To all those who have gone before me, who took the time and made the sacrifice to put their works into writing, I am grateful and indebted.   —*Michele*

PREFACE

IN MY EARLY YEARS as a student nurse enveloped in human suffering and tragedy, and later as a pediatric ICU nurse, I felt there was a connection between disease (and any human suffering) and God. I had no training, no religious roots or teachings, just a vague feeling that it was somehow connected. Since no one associated with medicine during those years ever talked about such things, I just thought about it...constantly.

Like so many before me, I couldn't conceive of a Creator who would allow such horror, ignore pleas and petitions, and afflict innocents, (The general human belief is that children are innocent and adults are not) much less someone who calls (Himself) LOVE.

Another thought that persisted throughout those early years was that there must be some common denominator of all disease. While the entire medical establishment was drowning in millions of various names, categories, symptomatology and treatments, I could not stop thinking that behind all the different presentations of all disease there was a root cause, whether communicable, degenerative, congenital or even trauma induced...something was working that we just didn't see. Perhaps because we were so entrenched in what we *did* see.

For a long time I pursued the study of God while still working in the medical field, believing that I was following two different paths at the same time...two different and conflicting paths. But I came to understand that the clear understanding of one would be the clear understanding of the other. And it would prove to be the resolution of the whole question of disease and human suffering.

Eventually I came into realizations that would alter my path forever. One was that medicine could never resolve the problem of human suffering, could never resolve the disease factor, could never answer the hard questions of suffering mankind. Why did this happen to me? Where did this come from? What might I have done to cause this? And what do I do now?

I also realized that religion and all the rhetoric concerning God and the origin of human suffering, had no consistent answers to the hard questions...and indeed, their explanations seem to solidify the necessity for suffering.

I remember years of watching as various clergy came to the hospital room to pray for healing for those agonizing under the weight of pain and fear and confusion. I saw that they also carried the same fear and confusion as the ones they came to pray for. Many prayed with one hand behind their back holding onto the doorknob for a quick escape.

And always ending the prayer with the famous "If it be your will, God, to heal them." Declaring for all the world to believe that it just might *not* be God's will for some to be healed!

I made up my mind that I would find my answers from God only, or die trying. Nothing I had heard so far made sense. It all seemed to severely contradict itself. The more I heard, the more I knew that no one really knew what was the truth. So I retreated from it all.

By this time I had left medicine, was an ordained minister, and then left that as well. The one thing that I didn't leave was the firm belief that God, Himself, would make it all clear. That there was an answer to it all and I would come to know it.

Up until now, disease has been the dreaded sentence upon innocent mankind, with little to no escape from its deadly grip. We have throughout the ages devised many palliative therapies for the myriads of ways that disease can afflict us, but these ways have by and large been just that, palliative and not curative. Nor have they offered anything but temporary reprieve, while we wait for the next wave of affliction to rear its head against us.

This mysterious and insidious enemy of health and wholeness has evaded man's most aggressive methods to curb, avoid or overcome it. It is relentless and is the root of all fears. The fear of disease and death has been referred to as the King of Terrors.

Modern medicine has 'come into its own,' offering a

dynasty of multi-million dollar diagnostic tools and devices...as well as chemical pharmaceuticals to overcome this elusive enemy, but sadly has failed in either protecting us from this experience or delivering us from its destruction. But has, in too many cases, even proven to exacerbate whatever the existing problem.

In blind desperation we began to attribute this horrible experience to God, our Creator. We imagined this as a punitive tool in His hands, reducing our concept of ourselves as being worthy of such torture, and He as being ruthless and beyond mercy in exacting our just reward. Our concept of God became equal to the distorted and convoluted appearances of the diseases themselves.

This was the prevailing thought which I was blindly entertaining when I had an experience which would challenge and change my entire perception of life, of God, of disease and the whole surrounding thought.

In 1970 my second daughter was born prematurely, with severe anoxia (lack of adequate oxygen) secondary to a premature lung disease, which left her hopelessly mentally retarded. I was advised to commit her to the "state school" for institutional care for the remainder of her life, thinking that I would be unable to handle such a severe situation at home. "She would never know the difference," they told me. The idea was unthinkable, so for months and years, alone and with no other visible means of help, I pressed on raising my two daughters.

It was during this time that a change occurred in my thinking which would lead me to begin to believe that there was indeed an avenue of escape from the tyranny of disease and affliction. *Instead of God being the progenitor of such experience, a new and more truthful understanding of Him would be the path of deliverance.*

Embracing these ideas, however faintly at first, eventually led to my daughter being completely healed of her mental prison and free to grow and develop normally into a thriving, lively adult. She enjoyed a normal childhood and adolescence and is today married, the mother of my first grandchild and a practicing attorney.

I have spent the rest of my life searching to understand how that happened and if there was a way to reproduce such healings. I knew without a doubt that I had nothing to do with my child's healing, at least not consciously. I knew that no one could tell me why she was healed or how it happened. Most of all was there a *principle* to be found, which if understood would enable people everywhere and under all conditions to also experience similar healings? I was assured by all my religious instructors that there was not. Indeed they said that not all people were supposed to be healed. And, as they reiterated the terrible power of evil in the earth, they assured me that it was the will of God that mankind suffer for their many offenses; to instruct them, to lead and guide them in a particular direction. They also declared that people often suffered for the offenses of others, as in children suffering for the sins of their parents.

In spite of these strange doctrines and through these years of searching, I began to witness unexplainable healings that soon began to happen with such frequency that I came to expect them. These could not be explained by medicine or science. I felt the presence of God in these healings, but still did not understand how they happened. Nor did I understand why people were experiencing disease to start with. Why did some people "get healed" and others not? Did some somehow qualify for their healing and others miss this? Who decided that, God, or the one suffering? Were we supposed to live with disease as part of the human condition? If so, why? And if not, how do we end this madness?

I eventually embarked upon a strange and new approach to healing that would later come to be called "alternative" or "holistic" for lack of a better category. Starting a center for healing in San Antonio, Texas, in 1975, I began to teach and to test this new approach while stretching to further understand it myself.

It combined a much more practical approach to health and personal responsibility in the care of our bodies, as well as a deep exploration and correction of our beliefs and understandings of life itself. I began to understand just how far we had strayed from the realities of life and of the true nature of God, why we are here and who we really are.

We found much to our joy and relief, that as these issues were cleared and elevated, and as we learned the proper care and maintenance of the body, our *expectation* of health and wholeness increased. This would invariably lead us into the *experience* of health and wholeness. In short, we learned to live outside the belief of the *inevitability* of disease. We learned that there are principles to healing, and more importantly, there are principles to living that will keep us free from the experience and effects of disease.

I paused after 40 years of healing practice to write a

book explaining and discussing these principles. My hope was to share my understandings with those who also seek recovery from affliction and are desiring of a new and more hopeful experience of life. My first book, "Of Monkeys and Dragons, Freedom from the Tyranny of Disease," outlines these principles, that are applicable to all of the distresses of the human condition, not singularly to disease alone.

The response to the book has been overwhelming, bringing hope and direction to those who find themselves floundering upon the shores of convoluted human ideology and its subsequent experience of dis-ease. It is for this reason that I desire to expand that work and to further explore the false images of the human consciousness that must be replaced with the Infinite Wisdom of the Mind of God.

So I turned my weary heart away from all that I knew, and began to learn to listen. And listen to learn. The discovery was beyond my greatest hopes and past anything I could have conceived of myself.

Now, convinced of the basic illegitimacy of disease to exist at all, convinced of the innocence of God as the progenitor of such events, and equally convinced of man's basic innocence...I declare for all the world to hear that man can be, and indeed was created to be, free from all disease and suffering. There is a way to be free from it all. There *is* "freedom from the tyranny of disease" and we can experience this now, regardless of our present circumstances.

I submit to you then this series of lectures and discussions as the basis for the unfolding of a new and more deliberate experience of Life, "on earth as it is in heaven."

WHO TOLD YOU...?

No one should ever have to hear, "Go home and get your affairs in order. There is no help for you." But thousands do hear those words every day. So much so that we have come to believe that this is the normal course of events and we should all expect that at some given time we will, in fact, be at that place in our own experience.

But if it is so normal, why do we resist it? Why do we run here and there to find help when we have been told that help doesn't exist? Why do we subject our bodies, our families and our finances to medical treatments that we know will not work?

I believe that one reason we resist what we are told is that we have not completely 'bought into' the idea that disease and destruction are really genetically or spiritually pre-programmed and a necessary part of life. I believe that down deep in the soul of every man, the truth about life and its purposes and expectations and realities, truly exists.

Here is the place where the everyday, *learned* beliefs collide with the *true, eternal realities*. So when confronted with disease, we react. We fight back. We declare that, in spite of what we know with our heads, our hearts say something different.

As a student nurse, way back in the early 60s, I saw plenty of this. I stood frozen as patients received their death sentences. I watched as the look of horror swept over their faces. I had the experience of seeing one man (I still remember his name) jump out of a hospital window to hasten the inevitable. And another one stretched out across his bed after drinking a cup of cyanide. Others simply and quietly acquiesced in silent submission to the words of those "who knew." After all, what could they do?

But then there were those, who after hearing the dreadful sentence against them, declared that there must be an answer. And they set out to find it. What made the difference, I always wondered? Why did some simply refuse to comply? Was it just defiance against an unjust sentence? Did they know something that I didn't know yet?

Admittedly, sometimes those folks didn't find their answer while they were still here. But I learned to admire them for not accepting those words as though they were the absolute word of God!

The medical profession mostly sneers at such conduct, believing that if they don't have the answer, then one simply doesn't exist. I am ashamed to admit that I was one of those, even going so far as to secure court orders to keep children under the "acceptable" medical care when their parents sought other avenues. I now refer to such behavior as "arrogant ignorance".

For awhile the whole thing was just miserable to me. I was confused and angry myself, evidently being one of those who defy an unjust sentence. I had a million questions and no answers, at least none that I trusted. But oddly enough I always had this vague feeling that someday I would find my answers. Some day we all would know, and then we would understand how to resist such tidal waves of anguish and destruction.

Gradually, and particularly after my daughter was healed, I began to believe beyond a doubt that we were supposed to challenge these situations. We were supposed to because they were absolutely illegitimate.

Who told us that pain and sorrow and suffering were necessary? Necessary for what?

That reminds me of the story of Adam and Eve. When confronted with the appearance of nakedness, Adam said to God, "I knew that I was naked and I was afraid." And God responded with, "Who told you that you were naked?"[1]

Who told us that we were weak and beggarly and lost and lacking? (That is what "being naked" really means... uncovered from the knowledge of our true identity). Who told us that we were so miserable and unworthy, and that only by consigning us to pain and weakness, suffering and despair could we ever be worthy again? Who told us all that? Who said that we needed disease or suffering in our human experience? Who said that we deserved it? Who first told us that we were of such a depraved nature that we drew upon us this experience in order to "balance the score" with God? Who told us that God required this? These are the words that I have heard from patients, clergy, and lay folks all of my life, when trying to explain the basic cause of human suffering.

Could the very accepting of such thoughts about God, about us, be what has allowed this suffering to exist?

Now the undeniable truth emerges out from under the rubble of prevailing religious thought...*God denies that we are weak and beggarly, sinful and needing to suffer to purify us from our miserable nature.* But it took me years and years to finally know that.

So let me take you step by step through what I have learned, and how it all unfolded to me. These new understandings finally corrected for me the beliefs that we have all held to. It's time to challenge these words and find the truth that was intended to free us from this whole miserable scenario.

Section I

INTRODUCTION

In this section we will look at the present collective human beliefs about disease and suffering in general. We will realize the futility of managing disease on a purely physical level and the self perpetuating error of seeing disease as having physical origins and causations.

We will introduce the whole issue of God as the progenitor of human suffering and the widespread religious beliefs that inculcated this concept into the hearts and minds of men. We will discover a higher truth, a purer understanding, concerning this issue and upon what basis we dare to look in a different direction. The hope and expectation of living beyond disease, of an entire change in the whole tragic picture, must by necessity begin with a new and sometimes radical correction in what we have come to expect without a pause or even a question. We will pause here to question.

And finally we will redefine health and disease, giving us common ground with which to begin our journey together.

Chapter One

A TARGET OUT OF REACH

Can we really live this life out of the reach of disease? Was it intended that we do so? Or has it been fore-ordained that we suffer disease, as so many now subscribe?

Where did it all start? Why did it all start? Is it coming from God as "just punishment?" Are we responsible? Did we "bring this on ourselves?" Most importantly, is there a way out of this horror...or is this a way to gain the glories of Eternal Life?

These are questions that must be explored in order for us to find our way out of this belief and subsequent experience. We must look at life from an entirely different perspective if we are to begin to experience life differently.

Is this possible? Absolutely. Not only possible but necessary if we are to become a target out of reach. So get ready for a journey of new understanding, one that will catapult you into a place of peace and a life without fear.

Probably a good place to start would be to examine some present prevailing beliefs about disease and health...about your body in general, about what actually constitutes your being and where it all began. We also need to understand some absolute truths about God...some that perhaps religion has distorted through ignorance and fear itself. We're going to find out why and where such human beliefs began and how that relates to the experience of disease and suffering.

One of the first prerequisites to this new understanding must be that we come to it with an open mind and a desire to honestly know the truth. We must come with at least a hope that there is another way to see life and that it will correct the present conditions. If we come clinging to our present beliefs, wrapping them around us like a shawl, defending and protecting the old... if we are loath to let go of anything already believed because of fear of change or an inordinate fear of "the God that we have created"...we will not gain much ground here.

It is impossible to approach this subject holding the same thoughts and beliefs and expect to get different results. That is why Jesus said, "You cannot put new wine into old wineskins."[1] First you must have a willingness to leave behind the old landmarks and trust that you are being taken by your hand and led to a greater place of thought, understanding and experience.

Perhaps you don't know God as ever-present Love yet: One you can abandon yourself to in trust and confidence. But by the time you have made this journey, you will. Remember if your old way of believing could have produced relief from your suffering, it would have done so by now!

To start, we must look at who we are, where we've come from and later on, why we are here. A knowledge of the source of our existence will determine how we view life, our bodies, and our health.

These questions are not new. Every age of mankind has asked them, each one offering their opinions and beliefs. With the scientific age dominating thought now, we have swung from believing that our beginnings were "in God" to having our beginnings in matter. Now we are simply the product of a random DNA, a genetic pool. We are matter from beginning to end.

For years, nearly a century or more now, it has been scientifically scoffed at to believe in a purely spiritual origin. As science became another "god that we created", any concept of a spiritual deity as our source and origin, and the governing force of our lives, began to be less popular.

With the social and sexual revolution in the 60's, man was loath to want to answer to a governing God, preferring to choose his own standard of living. Perhaps the real rebellion was more to prevailing religious teachings *about* God than to God Himself. But most people could not make the distinction, so the "baby got tossed out with the bath water."

In order to challenge disease and its right to exist at all, we need to find our way back to the idea of having a pure, spiritual origin of existence...*with our bodies as being simply vehicles of expression of our spirituality.*

If we are merely matter, random acts of chance, then so is disease (and every other human experience) a random act.

If this is the highest truth we can embrace, then we have nothing left to do but duck the blows as they appear! Which is pretty much what we have been doing anyway.

Medicine has taught us to look to matter for the cause of our infirmities. We examine our bodies to see what is causing our problems. We blame our age, our gender, our fathers and mothers. We blame our environment, the trees, the flowers, the grass, the seasons. We blame our habits of eating. We blame the water we drink, the air we breathe, and the soil which nurtures our crops.

We have become victims of the world we live in and the bodies we wear and the parents who loved and cared for us. We live in a victim mentality!

We have made everything a potential enemy. The most aggressive enemy is our own unpredictable body. And of course the only solution we are offered is a pill for every part of our body and everything that can go wrong.

This, you will agree, has become hysterical madness, with fear motivating our entire human experience.

Unfortunately, turning to God as both the progenitor of our life and the governing factor has become equally destructive. *And that is sadly because of the images we have been taught to believe about the nature of God.* These images have produced fear, dread and a *sense of separation,* both from God and from each other. They have made God unapproachable to us.

Religion has taught us our basic unworthiness and need to suffer to gain righteousness. It has given us a God that is terribly exacting in His nature and impossible to please.

Disease is then a result of, and a physical manifestation of, the confusion and defeat we feel... our inherent failure in the eyes of God. It is the result of being human. We have both created the experience and then created a reason for it to exist! How impossible then is it to approach God for healing with any degree of confidence, if we feel we have somehow earned this misery, and it is certainly "for our own good!"

Leaving both philosophies behind then, as both damaging and non-productive in our quest for a life without disease, let us press on to the truth about God and the truth about man. Let us *look to God* for our answers, turning away from "man's image of God" and his strange and convoluted ideas. Let us discover together what life was really intended to be and how to find it.

Disease is a physical manifestation of a belief. Not necessarily a personal belief, but a collective human concept...about God, about us, about life. These beliefs are so damaging as to cause the very dis-eases and suffering that we find now ruling our lives.

The good news is these beliefs can be challenged and corrected. With these new understandings will come new experiences in our lives and a freedom from such present enslavement.

It is my joy to share these with you now.

Chapter Two

CHALLENGING THE LEGITIMACY OF DISEASE

Disease is an illegitimate experience. Our fascination with it gives it the only power it has to exist. Our fear of it gives it the only power it has to overcome us.

Upon what basis do we think we have the right to challenge such a widespread belief and experience? And upon what basis do we dare to declare our God-given right to live above the grasp of such an experience?

Where did disease come from? How did it first appear and why? Is there a common denominator to all disease? And, if so, how will that understanding allow us to walk away from it?

This story is a perfect springboard to begin this discussion.

Only a few years ago a young man visited a spiritual practitioner. This is one who heals through the avenue of increasing awareness of one's spirituality and relationship with God. He announced that he had the dreaded disease of AIDS and was given only a few years to live. He did not request that the practitioner pray for his healing. He said that he knew that he was going to die and wanted only one thing before that happened. He wanted this man to help him to "know God." Not the strange and convoluted imagery of God that he fled from as a child. Not the usual patented answers that he heard throughout all his youth. But he wanted to really know God, if indeed God could be known. He was asking for an introduction, if you will, to his Creator, so that he could know Him personally. He wanted to understand life and the significance of it.

What was God's expectation of him? What was the meaning and purpose of this human experience? Who was God really and was it possible to know Him...to understand His character and nature, His thoughts and feelings?[1]

This practitioner was a gentleman who spent his whole life praying for people to be healed. But never had he heard such a request from one who had been given an imminent death sentence. Always people seek God for a favor, a blessing, a healing of some sort. Never had he met one who sought God simply out of a desire to know Him, no strings attached.

The healer was impressed with the sincerity and purity of this young man's heart and agreed to help him.

For two years they met twice a week and they studied and searched out the true knowledge of God.[2] They found that God, Himself, was eager to reveal to them His true nature and quickly responded to each prayer for understanding.

Their journey was buoyed with hope and an excited expectation that always accompanies a new and fresh discovery. Many old and well worn concepts were replaced with pure revelations of the nature of God and man's relation to that nature. *They found the mind and heart of God literally opened to them as they desired nothing less than truth.*

In the midst of this all consuming thought, the young man gradually became symptom free and later discovered that he had become HIV negative. He never asked for this, nor did he secretly hope for it. He realized that he did *nothing to earn it,* nor did he need to qualify by somehow making himself *worthy* for such an event to appear.

What he did realize was that he had come face to face with the true nature of God and this was the only possible result.

What did happen here? How and why did this happen? What do we need to glean from such an event? Most of all, is there a principle or a truth which if known and understood, would allow others to experience healing as well? Is there a *law* of healing or was this simply a roll of the dice and he came up with a lucky number?

To answer these questions...to understand what happened here and why...to find the hidden truths that caused this event to take place...and then to be able to reproduce such an experience, we must find out what he came to understand in his search for the true and living God and *how that knowledge could possibly cause such a shift in the human condition.*

This then is an account of the Law of Life, filtered through a new and brilliantly illuminated understanding of our Creator and Maker. A revelation of enlightenment which, when sought for with one's whole heart and soul, will heal, change and alter the course of one's life. The only prerequisite seems to be that we approach this with humility and a desire to know the truth more than we want to "be right." By this I mean that we gladly lay down our preconceived beliefs and opinions...all that we "know" and insist is right and correct...and let God Himself teach us about Himself.

How and why does that heal and correct the human picture? *Because as it turns out, we experience our lives according to our perception of God.* As that is corrected... our experience is corrected...without human effort or intervention.

Jesus said, "Blessed are the pure in heart, for they shall see (know, perceive) God."[3] And later we read the words of Paul, "To the pure, all things are pure."[4] That says to me that when we perceive purity of thought (truth) then everything appears pure, clean and whole.

Another scripture from II Samuel, chapter 22, declares, "With the merciful, thou will show thyself merciful. With the upright man, thou will show thyself upright. With the pure, thou will show thyself pure. But with the forward and unsavory, thou will show thyself to be hard and unapproachable."[5]

However we perceive God to be...that is how He appears to each one. As we allow that to be presented to us in a more pure and accurate understanding, then that, in and of itself, corrects the human appearance.

CHAPTER THREE

THE PARADIGM SHIFT

Not only must our understanding of the nature of God be corrected, but our acceptance of God's view of man, and indeed all of His creation, must therefore be rethought.

LET ME SHARE ANOTHER STORY with you to help you to better understand such a concept.

After my first book was published, I received hundreds of letters, emails and phone calls telling me that during the reading of the book, and without any particular human effort, they experienced healings...of their bodies, homes, marriages, relationships, finances, careers, etc. A perception shift was taking place as they read and the change in the human condition was the result of only that.

One such call I received came from a woman living in another Texas town who heard my weekly radio show, Living Beyond Disease, and asked that I support her through a surgery she was to have for the removal of a malignant breast.

She shared with me that she had no family or close friends with whom she felt comfortable during this very challenging time in her life. She would take a cab to and from the hospital. Although she was told that the cancer had spread beyond the margins of the breast, still in desperation, she agreed to the surgery.

The whole time she was telling me her story I was praying, asking God what I should say to her...what did He want her to know?

I told her that God did not see her with an affliction, but instead He saw only that which He had made and formed "after His image and likeness." That in the mind of God there was *never a change in that absolute truth.* Since however we live *"out from our vision of God and Life,"* the correction needed to come *personally* to her awareness as to what God actually saw.

We prayed together daily that she might see herself as God saw her, as He formed her out from His own perfection. I reminded her that "God saw everything that He had made and behold it was very good."[1] We looked up the Hebrew word, "good," and found that it meant, *perfect, undamaged, uninterrupted, and incorruptible.*

We spoke of the Law of Life that states, "Each seed reproduces after its own kind."[2] A carrot seed can only produce a carrot. An acorn can only become an oak tree. Each animal brings forth only after its own kind. And so it is with God. This is why it is so important to understand and to firmly believe that "It is He who hath made us and not we ourselves...the world and all that dwells therein."[3] Created by God, we must therefore learn to expect to appear in our lives only that which proceeds from the nature of God.

The day that she was to enter the hospital she bought a long stemmed, red rose and set it in a vase of water. She placed it beside her bed so that it would be the first thing that she saw upon awakening from the anesthetic. She prayed, "God let me be reminded, as I look upon the perfection of this rose, that it is the same beauty and order and wholeness that you see when you look at me. Let me see myself as you made me." That rose was indeed the first thing that she saw as she awakened from the surgery, and each time she looked at it she repeated her prayer.

Soon she was discharged from the hospital and she placed the rose on her bedside table at home. After a few days it turned to a dark, maroon color, its head was bent and the leaves were dry and brittle. She thought about throwing it away, but decided to put fresh water into the vase instead. Feeling a little foolish, she set the vase aside and went on about the daily business of recovering her strength. Days later she remembered the rose and upon approaching it she noticed, to her amazement, that there were now four new rose buds on that cut stem and each one was a different color!

She was ecstatic with the realization that God had indeed communicated to her in response to her request and that he had shown His delight in her. Needless to say the cancer never reappeared; she regained full health, a new career, the exoneration of a large previous debt and an incredible new insight into the heart and mind of God.

Disease is illegitimate. As a collective human thought, it is the outworking of a *heart which has beheld a sense of unworthiness*. Not only in itself, but has looked out to a world that it also judges as unworthy. The human heart attributes this unworthiness to a God who is disappointed with His creation, man. It believes that disease, as well as all human suffering, is a just consequence for having failed in the sight of God.

The collective human thought does not recognize itself as a reflection of the beauty and perfection of its source and origin, its Creator. Nor does it realize itself as being under the umbrella of His constant care. This is called having a "sin nature." The word *sin* here means *entertaining a sense of separation from the person and nature of God*. It always refers to a nature, a conscious awareness...not an action.

Although we have declared this negative judgment to be the nature of God, such a God never existed! Only in the minds of men who do not know God could such a distorted image of one so pure, so holy and so merciful ever exist. Disease is a result of a perception learned...a perception of God, man and life...and that perception, deeply erroneous. As this false imagery is healed and a new vision emerges, we will calmly stand up and walk away from whatever effect the misperception has caused. As we are corrected in our understanding, our whole world appears in Divine Order.

Soon mankind will shake off the grave clothes of such distortion of knowledge and finally be free to live and love and laugh without the fear and dread of disease. This is the appearing of the Kingdom (dominion) of God (goodness)... that which Jesus declared is, and has always been, already here.[4] Then it will be seen that the "earth will be filled with the knowledge of the Lord as the waters cover the sea."[5]

Our time is come...

For it is written that "all creation groans and travails in pain together waiting for the manifestation of the sons of God to appear."[6] It is then that the "lion and the lamb will lie down together."[7] "...and the voice of weeping shall be no more heard in the land, nor the voice of crying."[8]

Disease truly is illegitimate. God never created it, saw it, or designed any use for it. He has no good reason for it, never consigned man or any part of His creation to experience it.

As a matter of fact, once we know the nature of God we will realize that it is so contrary to His nature of order and perfection, that indeed it would be impossible for that to proceed out from Him at all. "He cannot deny Himself."[9]

Chapter Four

YOU SHALL KNOW THE TRUTH AND THE TRUTH SHALL MAKE YOU FREE

In seeking health or freedom from any oppression, you will find that it is not what you do or where you go, or to whom you reach out...but always *what you know*. What you are holding in thought. *Your basic belief system defines your expectation.* Your expectation defines your reality...or what you will experience.

So we read, "According to your belief (what you understand to be true) so let it be done unto you."[1] As thought is elevated and truth and wisdom replace the images and fears of disease, so will the experience be corrected.

This is a huge leap of understanding for some, as it certainly was for me. So I will do my best to take you step by step, as it was first presented to me, challenging as many old beliefs as possible, building a secure and whole new perception of life and foundation for living, until we all see it together. Once this groundwork is laid, we will discover how to use this new understanding to gain dominion over any presenting human challenge of life. We will still see life according to our understanding...but as that is changed, then so will our life change in accordance.

Many people today have made this transition of thought. Many are doing it right now. In fact, as civilization has progressed, these challenges to certain mind-sets are a necessary step in growth and progression. We see this in every field of human experience from religion to government, to inventions and discoveries of new technological advancements.

We are right now riding the crest of a whole new perspective of life. Let us explore this shift in thought without fear, but instead with certainty that we are being led step by step toward that which we all desire.

THE VEIL THAT BLINDS US

ALTHOUGH MANY YEARS and experiences have passed since I was first introduced to this new understanding of the cause of disease and the simplicity with which it can be removed, I will never forget how it first appeared.

In 1982 I found written in Isaiah, chapter 25: 7, 8…these words.

"There is a veil, a covering cast over all nations and all peoples of all nations. When that veil shall be removed, there will be no more pain, nor weeping, no sighing, no disease, no suffering, no death."

I probably stared at those words for hours, for days. Up until then I looked for the cause of disease on a purely physical plane. Physical effect must come from physical cause.

We have all been frozen in a world that looks for a cause for every ailment.

From the time we are born we are being examined for possible birth defects. We are watched for the possible appearing of hidden malfunctions. Later we are introduced to multitudes of drugs (immunizations) to keep us from getting childhood diseases. Diseases that are *expected* to happen to children.

Later we are instructed into the myriads of problems associated with our particular gender, age, and race. *All this convinces us of our inherent weakness, or vulnerability to disease.*

We learn to fear our bodies at a very early age. We have zero confidence in its ability to maintain health and wholeness. We are never taught the wonders of this body, only the sordid details of the failure of it to sustain life. We are encouraged to have it checked as often as we can to make sure it hasn't begun to fall apart yet. We grow to depend upon outside resources for the health and strength and wholeness of the body. Nothing within it can be trusted. Only a fool would trust their body. Only a fool would not get it checked. "Anyway it's just a matter of time until we get whatever we have been genetically programmed to get"...unless of course they find a way to reprogram our chromosomes for us.

So we look for those learned men and women who will save our lives; the same ones who convinced us to start with, that we were doomed to fall apart.

We have forgotten that it is "He who hath made us and not we ourselves."[1] We have forgotten that we are made in the "image and likeness of God."[2] We have forgotten that "He is our life and the length and strength of our days."[3] And we have forgotten that "He has created us for His glory."[4] We have forgotten from where we have come and to whom we belong.[5] And we have no idea why we are here...not really.

We are warned of seasonal diseases, causing us to fear the earth that we were given to live in and enjoy. We are afraid of the flowers that bloom and the wind that blows. We have forgotten that these things were made for our enjoyment. We have forgotten that they were made by the same substance and came from the same origin that we were! We have forgotten that *we all live by the same life!* To fear something that is also made by the same life that made you, is to fear your own life!

We are given statistics and grave sentences upon us around every corner, just for being alive. We are told what to eat. What not to eat...and that changes weekly.

We are told in essence that we live under the Law of Chance and Probability. A roll of the dice. And that we are personally responsible for our lives, even though we have no idea what it needs or how to do it. The instructions are too conflicting.

Then, when we fall apart, "we have only ourselves to blame!"

I can honestly tell you after taking care of sick folks for over 40 years, that those who become obsessed with their health and the personal care and maintenance of their bodies, no matter how much they fret over it, get just as sick as those who don't go down that road. Learning the wisdom of the basic care of the body is great, but doing it out of fear is counter-productive.

So this is the scientific brilliance of this human age. This is their take on the issue of disease and life.

In enters religion and the learned wisdom of the sages. "Yes," they say, "God made us. But that is no assurance that we will remain in the condition that He created." Or they would have to admit that God makes imperfections. And since God is perfect and we are made by Him and in His image...and yet we fall apart, it must be something we have done to deserve this or to have made this happen.

I have stood by thousands of sick people who have been told that the cause of their sickness is their own doing. They cry, they repent...again and again...and still no relief. Can you imagine how isolated they must feel from others and how abandoned they feel by God? Who in the earth could get well with this going on in their hearts and minds?

Disease, they say, comes from sin and every one of us fall into that category. Even your babies. Even your children. Can anyone honestly accept this? Many folks have spent their lives serving God, doing everything they have learned to "please God" and still succumb to disease. How do we explain all this?

I am reminded of the story of Job in the Bible. Job was a "righteous man who loved God and hated evil."[6] He was kind, benevolent and full of graciousness to everyone. He was wise and well loved. He enjoyed enormous wealth and blessings. He fulfilled "all the demands of the law" to please God and atone for any sin he might have committed. He "sacrificed" day and night, not only for himself but also for his children, in the event that they might sin.

Even so, horrible hardships befell Job. His crops failed, his livestock all died. Soon his children all died as well. Finally his health failed and his body became covered with sores and painful boils. Those who once loved him and respected him now ran from him. He was considered to be "cursed of God." Hmmmm...sound familiar?

The religious leaders of the day surrounded him with declarations of "hidden sins" he must have committed. When he denied this, they accused him of self righteousness.

Finally the day came when God revealed Himself to Job. He spoke to him and declared His nature to him. He *opened the eyes of Job* and caused him to see things that Job never saw before. *Upon seeing something new,* Job was forever changed...his health and all his wealth and possessions were reestablished. He had many more children and he was once again looked upon with great admiration, position and leadership.

What happened?

Job saw something.

The veil was removed and he saw something that he never saw before.

And that very *seeing* caused a change in the entire physical, visible picture.

෨

You see, nothing needed to be changed or fixed or healed. No "cause" needed to be found. Only the veil of perception needed to be removed!

Suddenly I realized that the Bible was a book about man's progressive *seeing*. Step by step man was being introduced to God, and to who they were and where they came from. Many years and generations of progressive unfoldment...each new understanding giving a clearer picture of God and erasing the old misconceptions.

Job declared, when his eyes were opened, "I cover my mouth for I have spoken of you that which I knew not. I have heard of you by the hearing of my ears, *but now I see you.*"[7]

What was it that Job saw? What was it that changed his life forever and restored to him his health, his life?

Whatever it was, it stopped the mouths of all those who professed to Job that they knew God and the reasons for his afflictions. Whatever it was, it was life changing and capable of causing Job to live without the fear of disease, without the fear of God causing disease, or with the need to please God in order to be safe from suffering. It completely altered his understanding and because it did, his life would never be the same.

Remember that Isaiah tells us that when the veil is lifted we will never experience disease or suffering. Now we no longer look to our bodies as weak and vulnerable or the cause of disease at all. Now we can rest in the gentle trusting of our body, which God has made and given to us to use during our stay here in this "parenthesis in eternity." Now we don't have to fear it, check it, give it to strangers to poke and prod, pour chemicals into and cut things out of it.

We just need to see something different!

Now we don't need to fear the earth and all that grows and lives and roams upon it. Now we can appreciate how a "new heaven and a new earth" will appear to us. We only need to see something different.

Now we don't have to fear a God of judgment and wrath and vengeance. A God so impossible to please and equally impossible to run from. We don't need to live under a cloud of self loathing, condemnation and unworthiness. We can see ourselves as beautiful and "wonderfully made."[8] We only need the veil lifted and everything will appear differently.

So what about this veil? And how is it lifted?

It took eight years of steady praying and wondering, asking and listening. Somewhere during that time another story jumped out at me and once again drove deep into my heart the same message over and over again.

CHAPTER SIX

JOHN 9

THIS IS A STORY ABOUT A MAN who was blind from his birth. The story took place during the ministry of Jesus.

The first thing that we read here is the followers of Jesus asking why this man was born blind. They wanted to know if it was his sin or the sins of his parents. Jesus answered in one word, "Neither."

Then he began to heal the man, "So that the glory of God would be revealed."

He made clay with spit and dirt from the ground and covered the man's eyes. This was to signify that it is the "earthbound thought" that must be removed. Only that which has been taught with human understanding needs to be uncovered. The idea that we came from dust needed to be cleared from the eyes of his heart.

He then told the man to go to a pool called "Sent" and wash the covering from his eyes. He did so and was instantly healed.

As soon as the man realized that he was "sent" by God to this human condition with purpose and intention, he was healed. No more was he simply a result of human will, a chance happening. He was sent by God! He was filled with a sense of Divine purpose! He was not a random DNA at all, but instead a deliberate act of God! Any sense of separation from God, from his source and origin, was removed. He realized he was *one* with the Spirit and purpose of God.

As the glory of this revelation dawned upon him, all sense of unworthiness, all belief in the necessity for suffering and affliction vanished. He was free to accept and experience his inherent wholeness.

Later, when interrogated by the religious leaders of the day, he was asked to deny this healing. This was way beyond their religion of Law and it frightened their security. They kept asking him if he was really the man who was born blind...and finally he answered them by saying, *"I am."*

This "I Am" was the same description that God gave to Moses at the burning bush, so those who heard him threw him out of the synagogue, believing him to be a heretic. But he knew who he was and of what Spirit he was. Every bit of the old identity was gone and he declared his oneness with God and with the purpose of God.

I used to wonder why so many folks were blind during the time Jesus was healing and teaching. Now I realized that it was speaking of the blindness *to who we are and why we have come.* It was the healing of the *sense of separation* from our real identity. That was, and still is, the blindness that Jesus spoke of when he said, "Those who know they are blind, shall see. But those who profess to see, shall remain blind."[1]

Once again the veil was lifted and what was seen healed and changed a life forever. Gone was the human sense of unworthiness and separation from our good. Gone was the sense of lack and limitation. Gone was the human struggle and failure. Gone was the distorted understanding of the God that humanity created...forever replaced with the true and everlasting God of Eternal goodness.

CHAPTER SEVEN

EVERY BIT WHOLE

ANOTHER PERHAPS MORE FAMILIAR STORY took place at what is called the "last supper" that Jesus had before his crucifixion.

The disciples had gathered in the *upper room*... signifying an *elevated understanding* was to be revealed that night.

At some point Jesus took a towel that he had wrapped around himself and began to wash the feet of his disciples. Although this was a common custom, they were uncomfortable with this since he was the Master and teacher and they, His students.

When it came to Peter's turn he protested and would not allow Jesus to wash his feet. Jesus said, "If I do not wash your feet, you will have no part with me." So poor Peter, confused but not wanting to be left behind said, "Then wash all of me!" But Jesus told him that it was not necessary that the rest of him be washed, because *"He was already every bit whole!"* Only his feet needed to be washed![1]

This once again points to the accumulation of dust and grime picked up as we travel along this earthly season of existence. It is referring to the human condition, the human thought that blinds us to who we are and why we are sent here. We pick up so much of the collective dirt and dust of strange theology, physiology and psychology that must be washed away if we are ever to see and know and understand.

It is not that our identity is changed...not at all. Only that now we are able to see...with no covering, no veil, *to what has never changed.* When this event appears and we are made aware of who and why we are here...no disease, no fear of disease will ever find a place within us again. We will then realize that no human effort is needed to fix something that is broken...for we are and have always been "every bit whole!"

We are not who and what we have been told since birth. We are no longer the victims... no longer living out from a sense of lack and fear of loss.

We have risen to a level of awareness that transcends the man made laws of existence. Now we live by the Law of perpetual Life.

Chapter Eight

ATMOSPHERES OF THOUGHT: LEVELS OF CONSCIOUS AWARENESS

"For my thoughts are not your thoughts, neither are my ways, your ways. For as the heavens are higher than the earth, so are my ways higher than your ways and my thoughts higher than your thoughts." Isaiah 55:8, 9.

THERE ARE LEVELS OF UNDERSTANDINGS and attitudes, a "sense of awareness" from which we function and live, without thought or question. I call these "atmospheres of thought."

As the history of man has progressed, our understanding of our lives, our relationship to our world, who we are, where we've come from and why we are here, also has progressed and elevated.

Historical scholars give accounts of the sociological and religious changes of thought throughout generations that finally gave way to new beliefs and new levels of human consciousness. As our understandings change and evolve, we begin to live our lives out from new atmospheres of thought, often resulting from wars, climatic events, widespread disease, or even disappointing religious leaders, leading to revolts and new revelations of God. Whatever the catalyst, these alter the present consciousness and open the way for new and purer understandings, elevating man to greater social awareness and also deeper understandings of God and their relationship to their Source.

We are right now being carried into a whole new perspective of human thought, particularly in the arena of health and religion (man's view of God).

And as in any of the previous historical accounts of such radical paradigm shifts of understanding, there will be those who resist the change. Usually they do so fearing the upheaval of their own personal security.

But there are those, nevertheless, who reach for a higher awareness, a better way of living that comes from a purer understanding. Among those are they who found that the present accepted beliefs of both disease and disease management are simply not working. They also have discovered that the present accepted view of God and particularly as it relates to human suffering doesn't fit anymore either. It's like a shoe that becomes too tight. Finally you can't walk another step without taking the old shoe off and finding another.

Let's explore these shifts of thought. We are looking for the relief of suffering and fear of disease. We must either understand why God allows or designs such misery or discover another concept of God. The only other alternative is to acquiesce to such a nightmare and continue to chase our tails trying to learn to cope with our diseases, or drown in the drugs now being used to squash the symptoms, only to create new and worse problems than before. Someone once told me that the clearest definition of insanity was to continue doing the same thing you have been doing and somehow expect a different outcome! To realize a different conclusion, we must begin with a different premise.

A new experience must begin with a new thought. A new revelation. A paradigm shift in understanding. An elevated atmosphere of thought.

I've said this already, but it needs to be said again and again... then I will probably need to spend the rest of my life trying to explain it. *We are experiencing our life (for good or ill) according to our personal understanding of God.* As we understand God, so we see ourselves and our relationship to God and to our world.

To be free of disease, and even the very dread of it, is the way we were intended to live. It is possible right here, right now.

It will not come, however, by dealing with the problem on a physical level. We can arrest symptoms in certain cases by doing something on a physical level, but we will never be assured that it, or something else, will not return. In other words, *we cannot change our expectation, our consciousness, by taking a pill.* Just because a problem appears as a physical one doesn't mean the solution must come by simply dealing with it physically.

To be free of disease, we must no longer fear it. We must no longer do things or take things to avoid it. We must no longer *see* it as a part of our experience. We must somehow see ourselves as beyond the grasp of such experience. This is not going to happen by anything that we do...*but by what we know*. And that *knowing* can only come when we see something differently.

There must be an eternal, legitimate reason for our hope, otherwise we are simply trying to eliminate something by an act of the human will. And that never works.

I should have a dollar for every patient who has sat across my desk and with gritted teeth declared, "I'm going to lick this!" or, "No disease is going to take my life!" My heart melts at the sound of their words, because unless there is a new and higher understanding birthed within their souls, their act of self-will will never save the day.

So it's not so much what we do, *as what we know*. Let's look at what we have known that might have resulted in this human experience called disease and suffering and then let's look at life from an entirely new perspective.

CHAPTER NINE

AN ELEVATION IN UNDERSTANDING

$\mathbf{M}$Y FIRST CONSCIOUS THOUGHT OF GOD as it related to human suffering was as a young pediatric ICU nurse. My days and nights were filled with children and babies deformed, diseased, suffering and separated from their homes and parents.

Frightened beyond description and utterly isolated from any measure of safety and security, these little ones were subjected to horrors of treatments that defy description. Most of the time the treatments were so much worse than the diseases. This was the condition, and probably still is, of my daily workplace.

Why does this exist? That question persisted relentlessly for years with no answer in sight and with no one I knew to turn to.

The prevailing religious answers were more unacceptable and horrible than the diseases that I came to hate so much.

Was this what God was? The progenitor of human

horrors? Or at least someone who *could* fix them but might not *want* to?

And where did such an image of God first appear...and why?

And so went my earliest introduction to God. Someone very far away, who sent us here, left us to figure it out and then punished us for not getting it right.

I found myself fighting for the lives of my patients *by trying to stand between them and this awful God*. I wondered why the children and babies suffered so. Were they being punished for the sins of their folks? Or was God afflicting the kids to make the parents suffer more? Kind of like the horrible dictators of so many countries who torture the kids to punish the fathers. It sounds so horrible now, but still so many people hold to that thought, having no other to replace it. They still ask me if this is happening to their child because of something that they did. No different than what I used to believe.

Just a few years ago a family brought to me a young child diagnosed with a malignant brain tumor. They confided to me that their family and church told them that she was sick because they were pregnant with her before they were married. They prayed and cried and repented, but she was still sick. Once they were able to eliminate such a concept of God from their frightened minds and replace it with one of *uninterrupted, unconditional Love...unearned, and always present...* the child was able to experience healing. In only a few short months every evidence of the disease was gone, never to reappear.

At the same time another mother brought her son with the exact same diagnosis, but she never for an instant believed that God had anything to do with this experience. *Instead of spending time trying to figure out why this happened,* she held to the thought that he was *made in the image and likeness of God,* and that God "made him to be strong and healthy, to grow into a strong and healthy and happy man."

She was clear that God was Love. Not a God who loved, but Love Itself. It was always a forgone conclusion in her mind that this experience was *as unacceptable to the nature of God* as it was to her. She never looked for a cause, but denied it on the basis that it was totally illegitimate, having never been sent from God.

She told her son that he was made by God to be whole and complete, strong and healthy. She repeated it almost hourly, day after day. They soon discovered that the tumors were gone and they also never reappeared. That was over eight years ago.

I remember an incident that happened when I was on an adult ward as a student nurse. I miscalculated a drug dose and overdosed a lady causing her blood pressure to crash. I stood against the wall in her room, out of the way of what seemed like hundreds of doctors and nurses running in and out trying to fix what I had done. I was terrified, paralyzed with the thought that she might die. It was the first time in my life that I ever remember praying. I ran from her room down to the chapel, knelt down and begged God not to let her die. I promised Him everything and anything if He would please not let her die. I bargained with everything including my own life. All night long I ran back and forth from her room to the chapel. Finally she was stabilized and we all went home.

I wondered at that whole scenario with God. Could He be coerced? If I cried hard enough and begged long enough, could I change His mind? It was all I had, so for years and years that was my approach to God. As I found myself standing between God and the sick and suffering people, I imagined that I was their friend, approaching a hard and angry God, trying to get Him to change His mind and let them be free. God was something like Pharaoh or Stalin in my mind, but with this proviso...He could be made to change His course of action if I worked hard enough at it. The fact that I read, and was being told, that God was Love might as well have been another language to me. It never found a place of comprehension in my mind. In Bible school I was told that God had to punish man for being so terrible. But then He sent Jesus to suffer and die in our behalf. He then sent us to pray to Jesus, which would often result in God changing His mind. That was their best understanding of Love. A discussion that I have saved for the last section of the book.

Even after I began to see so many healings in my career, and in my family, I still held to some scrambled, convoluted remnants of the old ideology of the nature of God. The God that man created! I had nothing new to put into its place.

∂

As the years progressed I saw so many hard evidences that God is really Love. I saw that God is the absolute and only Life of us and of all creation, and is as near as the air we live in. My misperceptions of God finally gave way to the realization that God is only pure Goodness, eternal Wisdom, ever present Counselor, and that God holds all that He has made in perpetual Divine order, by Intelligence and Understanding.

When it was all said and done and there were no more doubts, *it still came to a decision, a choice to believe this and live by this understanding.*

After all, we made a choice to believe the raw, adulterated version of the nature of God for centuries…

Why not choose again?

CHAPTER TEN

THE CREATIVE INFLUENCE OF THOUGHT

How does what we "know" make something appear? How does thought translate into visible manifestation? In other words, how will a change in my understanding, (therefore my expectation) cause something different to appear or happen?

We are so entrenched in "western thought" which teaches us that cause and effect are always on the physical realm.

Notice that whenever something happens we immediately state a physical reason for its appearing. Such as, "my head hurts; must be stress, or must be not enough sleep, or sinuses, or barometric pressure, or eye strain," etc.

Take an automobile accident. Immediately we blame ourselves, speeding, the other guy, the weather, the road conditions, etc. We are always looking for the *physical* cause of every effect.

Look at how we view disease. Every symptom, every

appearance of dysfunction has some physical cause. Even if what we are saying is absurd and idiotic, we hold to our beliefs.

We believe that microorganisms, though unseen, have the power to overcome health and wholeness. What is the problem with that belief? Just that we are giving more power to microorganisms than we are to the Life within us. You see, we have within us an immune system that is designed to keep out all foreign invasion. It is our protective system. It is governed by the intelligence and wisdom of the Spirit of Life that motivates it. To fear being overcome by foreign influence is to deny the presence and power of this Life energy, or Spirit of Life within. *We are giving more power to that which is created than to the Creator who made it!*

We believe that a child, because he is small and dependant upon us for survival, is weak and vulnerable to many and varied "childhood diseases."

We believe that someone is an alcoholic because their father was.

We believe that if you get your head wet, you will get a "cold."

Years ago we said that everything was caused by an unseen virus, now the new fad and fashion of thought is that everything is genetic in origin.

Always we must find a cause and always that cause must be from something physical.

Now lately we blame everything on stress; anxiety and its effect upon the adrenal system.

So we are reduced to battling diseases, as well as all human problems, *by avoiding the cause.* This creates a lifetime of fear. We fear everything that life has for us, believing that it all has the propensity to hurt us. Including our own bodies.

We fear the environment, nature and the changing seasons. We fear each other. We fear our present image of a God that dropped us into this maze of danger and left us here.

Or worse, we fear our present image of God, Who deliberately caused or allowed this to happen to us because we "needed it", "deserved it" or unwisely "chose it."

In short, we blame everything we can think of for our present circumstances and therefore fear everything we know.

But there is no human condition, regardless of how severe, how it manifests, how long one has experienced it, how deadly the world views it to be, *that will not yield to a change in our present understanding of Life, and of the source and origin of all Life.*

Everything that appears begins with an accepted thought, belief, an understanding. And it all comes from living in a specific level of conscious awareness. The one that is described here is, of course, called the human consciousness.

With no thought to the contrary, we believe what others believe. We think what others think, we expect what others expect, and so we experience what others experience.

We see what we are taught to see. We know what we are taught to know.

Unless we make a concerted effort to "see" beyond,

unless we are willing to find the "unfindable," search the unsearchable, know the unknowable, we will remain stuck in this human consciousness and spend our lives dodging the problems that arise.

That is what prompted Albert Einstein to declare, "No problem can be solved by the same consciousness that created it." We will never find the answers or solutions to our human problems within the confines of the human intellect, human will, human brilliance or human wisdom (oxymoron).

Centuries of reliance upon science, medicine or psychology, should have given us the clue here. We now experience far more diseases, far greater mental disorders than ever known in the history of man. The law of *chance* rules us. That is, whatever happens to happen will be our lot. No matter how hard we try to avoid human misery, we are still living under the proverbial *roll of the dice.*

The only solution is an escape from the human consciousness into another Mind, another thought, another realm of experience. A higher atmosphere of thought.

Can we do this while presently living within the confines of the human experience? We *must* do this while presently living within the confines of the human experience! Otherwise there is no hope of changing the human experience.

I will tell you of my first awakening to this *higher,* more perfect realm of thought. Those of you who have read my first book, *Of Monkeys and Dragons,* will remember that my early years were fraught with misery and disasters. I found my hope by escaping into an awareness of God as my helper, One who would love and care for me and my children all the days of my life. Consequently I prayed and sought God continually, both for my family and my patients who were suffering from the ravages of disease beyond human description.

I read and believed that God would deliver us from our present circumstances, if we prayed enough and somehow *pleased* God. And even if we failed to please God, we could always be forgiven and therefore still be cared for by God.

On this level of understanding, I found God to be faithful and merciful. I saw many hundreds of *healings* for both my family and my patients.

I also read and understood that I was being commissioned to heal those who were sick and suffering. I wanted to do that, and believed that the way to accomplish this was *to ask God to do it* and hope He would.

I read how Jesus healed the multitudes and knew that I was to do the same. But I never really knew *how* he did those healings, nor how to imitate them myself.

Have you ever felt like there was just one more piece to the puzzle that you hadn't seen and it was just one inch from your ability to reach it?

In 1984, after years of witnessing so many healings for so many people, I began to notice that many, once healed of horrible situations, were being killed in accidents or entrenched in problems worse than those they experienced previously. In other words, their healing was wonderful for the moment, but seemed to be unable to lift them into a higher realm of awareness that would keep them safe and secure from trouble. I began to feel like the proverbial mouse whirling about all day long on my wheel...going nowhere.

Why was I fighting so hard for victory over something that only would find a way to appear again and again? Was there no permanent solution to disease? Was there no way to live above the very reach of it altogether? Was it even possible? Were we supposed to? Or was this, as we are so often taught from childhood, a way for God to deal with a creation gone astray?

One day while sitting at my desk interviewing a patient, and with all these thoughts bouncing about in my head like a ping pong ball, I heard what I have come to know as the voice or impulse of the Spirit of God in my mind asking this question,

"How do you suppose Jesus healed the man with the withered hand?"[1]

This is a story, recorded in the book of Luke, of a man whose congenitally deformed hand was healed by Jesus, in the temple, on the Sabbath day. He simply told the man to stand, stretch out his hand and it was changed to look like the other hand in that instant.

In response to the question, it occurred to me that I didn't know *how* he did any of the healings that I read about. There didn't seem to be any pattern of *how* they were done. On the surface each one seemed different from the others. So after what felt like an eternal thirty seconds or so, I answered, "I really have no idea." The answer was quick and definite. "He never saw it withered!"

Whoa! I thought. Hold on here! "He never saw it withered?"

Then what *did* he see?

He saw the eternal perfection of that which was created by Eternal Perfection!

I suddenly felt like the Mad Hatter, spinning out of my orbit of thought into wherever this new thought took me.

What then did Jesus see? He saw what God sees. And what does God see? He sees what He has made, formed, created. He does not see what we have believed or created by our distortions, confusions and misunderstandings. He sees what He knows is true. Only that which has come forth from Himself.

Referring once again to the verse in Genesis that declares, "Each seed comes forth from its own kind," we know this is true. All of creation tells us this is true.

This is true of God and that which God forms from His own being as well. Perfection can only create perfection. Beauty, order, harmony and goodness can only bring forth beauty, order, harmony and goodness.

Jesus *had found his way into the mind or thought of God.* He had found that we truly are made "in the image of Him who made us." He believed it so much that he saw the reality of it *right where the opposite seemed to appear to mortal thought.*

Now it suddenly occurred to me that what I had been doing for so many years…indeed what the whole world was doing… was to first *agree* with this error of thought, that we were weak and vulnerable with a propensity towards suffering, and that there must be a "good" reason for it all...and then appeal to God to change it!

I was looking at the veil of human misperception, *calling it true*, and then trying with drugs, surgeries, alternative programs, prayer, fasting, pleading, "energy work," yoga, and anything and everything imaginable, to correct what was only present and visible to the human belief system...*but never present to God.*

The answer was clear, that to find the Mind of God...that is to escape into another, higher atmosphere of thought and knowledge, was the permanent answer to the human dilemma.

To see through and beyond what was visibly appearing into what never changed was the answer.

My favorite scripture in Ecclesiastes reads, "I know that whatever God does shall be forever. Nothing can be added to it nor anything taken from it. And God does it that men should honor Him alone."[2] In spite of such words of truth and wisdom, we still create a lifetime of changeableness and insecurity by our lack of understanding of such wisdom.

A major portion of the human veil was lifted for me that day. My entire understanding was altered. Now, instead of trying to fix problems that seem to exist and torment people, I strove and prayed *to see as God sees, know only what God knows* and thereby honor the eternal truth that never changes. The word here is *immutable.* It means never changing and is a permanent attribute of that which is eternal...God, the source of us all.

Now I wanted to see everything through the eyes of Truth and Wisdom and Life and Love.

But one question yet remained. The Proverb says, "As a man thinks in his heart, so is he."[3] How does what one sees, knows and truly accepts as true reality, cause a change in and on the human scene? How does thought produce and correct reality? How does belief find its way to visible expression?

Remember we are talking about a "collective" human thought, not necessarily an individual thought. This collective human thought, out from which we have our experiences, is what we have been referring to as an "atmosphere of thought."

As we "collectively" think in our hearts, we become. *Until that image is transcended by the appearing of a higher atmosphere of thought,* we will continue to see ourselves and feel about ourselves, only from whatever image we have been told or thought.

For instance, a child will develop into whatever kind of person that he has been made to believe that he is. Our image of ourselves is formed by that which is projected onto us from those in our experience. If we are made to believe that we are capable of anything we desire, our image of ourselves will be quite different from that of a child who is made to feel he is constantly wrong and incapable of doing right.

A criminal personality is one who is "acting out" his image of himself. If he were to see himself differently, he would begin to act differently.

A scholar has that thought within himself that knows he is capable of having an understanding of even the most complex issues of life. That expectation is the soil out from which the plant grows and flourishes.

When someone is chronically ill, we can continue to deal with the physical appearances of the symptoms, or we can begin to deal with the image of being weak, fragile, vulnerable and victimized, sinful and worthy of such suffering. We can begin to deal with man's perception of the inevitability of suffering.

This idea of living out our lives according to our image of ourselves is really critical.

Since the beginning of written historical accounts, man has believed himself to be worthy of suffering and the more we experienced this phenomena, the more entrenched was this belief.

Now I realized that faith went a heck of a lot further than just the words of our mouths or the churches we belonged to. This was going to take a lot of prayer and a lot of changes in thought and perception. This was going to be a radical shift into another Mind.

The good news is that it is the *will and purpose* of God that we live our lives according to *His* image of us and not the ones that we have adopted for ourselves. From the beginning it was intended that we experience a "oneness" with this Mind, knowing what it knows and seeing what it sees. So we don't have to struggle to enter into it, as though trying to overcome God's reluctance to share this. We don't have to reach out for it. We don't have to beg or somehow qualify for it. We cannot earn it, for it is not for sale! We only need to desire to see it and it appears. No struggle, just definite intention and desire. It takes a deliberate act of *receiving* and that becomes possible when we are convinced that it was, and is, *our mind* as well and we have really never been separated from it...although it certainly seemed so for a long, dark time. ("For we have the mind of Christ.")[4]

༄

One more startling discovery appeared to me during that same time frame.

I was reading my Bible one evening and came upon a story in the book of Genesis. It was the story of Jacob, one of the twin sons of Isaac. For years Jacob worked for his uncle Laban, tending his herds and his land. He married both of Laban's daughters and had two concubines as well. (Acceptable for those days) Jacob had eleven sons at the time of this story, and one daughter.

He felt that it was time for him to break away from Laban and start his own life by returning to his native land. He wanted to care for his own family and begin to build his own resources. He asked for a portion of Laban's herd to get him started, citing that it was he who actually built up Laban's herd to be what it was to that day! So Laban offered Jacob "all the speckled, spotted, and brown cattle of the herd."

Since they were few in number, Jacob decided to increase them and this is how he did it.

Jacob knew that every morning and every evening the cattle came up for watering. So he took a poplar tree and cut off several branches. With his knife he cut the branches to appear speckled and spotted and he placed these speckled and spotted branches into the watering trough for the cattle to look at as they drank morning and evening, knowing that they would then conceive *only that which they saw*. There was no small contention when Laban realized that Jacob was leaving with much more than Laban was being left with! It says that Jacob's herd excelled that of Laban's many times and he took what was promised and left.[5]

Even then the truth was a clear principle of life. Jacob knew that what we see is truly what we get! What we "hold in thought" is what we will create in experience.

I had never heard anyone even so much as mention that story in all my years of Bible study and I certainly had no understanding, myself, of how that happened.

How could just looking at something cause it to appear as a physical entity? What is it about "seeing" or envisioning something that actually creates it in the physical world? How far does the power of the imagination, or imaging, really reach?

Soon after that, as Jacob was traveling back to his home land, he got a message that his twin brother was coming for him with the intention of killing him. Jacob had left his home years before because he had deceived his brother and stolen from him, and now he feared for his life. It looked like the day of reckoning had finally come. Jacob was so terrified and sure of his imminent destruction that he separated himself from his family and sent them another way to protect them.

In desperation Jacob prayed all night. It says that he wrestled with an angel (messenger of truth), signifying that his struggle was internal. He was pulling down strongholds of belief and allowing a new and clearer understanding to emerge.

When the "day broke" (the light of truth revealed) he had reconciled his heart with the heart of God!

Later when his brother approached with an army of men, Jacob looked at him and "saw the face of God."[6] No more did he see the face of anger and hate, of revenge and retaliation. His mind was clear, his vision was pure. He saw that which never changes. He saw God appearing in the form of his brother. *He saw that God is never separated from that which He has created.* He saw what we would *all see* if we chose...*God being manifested as His creation, and all creation defining and declaring the glory of God!*

Herein is the Mind of God.

And as always proves to be true, the invisible, unseen world of the Glory of God appears as soon as we are able to *see* it. Such is the definition of faith, the ability to see what is not visible, thereby allowing the unseen reality to appear.

His brother ran to greet him and kissed him and forgave his injury to him. They were reconciled at that moment and forever.

Once again it is not so much what we do that makes the difference, but what we know, what we choose to see with our hearts and our understanding. Perception creates reality.

~

The immutability of God, and consequently the immutability of that which proceeds from this source, is most important for us to grasp. This is one of the most obstructive misrepresentations of God that exists now.

Contrary to popular belief, *God is not reactive*. God is unchangeable and constant. God is not a man who watches and judges what he sees and decides to reward or punish accordingly...like Santa Clause. God is Spirit and that Spirit dwells in perpetual truth, and *is* perpetual truth. That truth is perpetual goodness. As we are able to come into agreement with this eternal truth of the present perfection of God and man, we will benefit by it. If we are stuck in the belief of a God who rewards and punishes, goodness that must be earned, then we will continue to miss the benefit of this truth. It is *we* who vacillate and are reactive to every thought and appearance that we perceive. It is we who choose to enter into or remain outside of the blessings. It is we who feel unworthy to receive such perpetual goodness. It is we who judge ourselves, then believe that judgment arises within the heart of God.

Because we judge that God is "man-like," and therefore subject to being reactive and changeable, we pray and appeal to Him to do things and to change the course of our human events. But God is constant and never changes.

So what must we do? We must leave behind that which we see, that which we fear is true, and allow ourselves to enter the atmosphere of thought which never changes and never knows anything but perpetual goodness. *We must enter into the heart and mind of God.* When we reach that sense of awareness all things in the visible world of expression will appear changed.

Now our prayers are for understanding and a correction of thought, rather than an appeal for change in the world of events.

Chapter Eleven

ENERGY OF LIFE...SPIRIT OF LIFE

T HOUGHT IS ENERGY. Just as light is energy. Since sound is also energy, that makes our words to be energy, as well. Even though science declares this to be so, it is difficult for some to understand.

We Westerners are so opaque in our thought that something like this is difficult to grasp. To tell the truth, I still can't grasp the idea of sound coming through my radio, much less pictures and sound coming through my television set. I am amazed that we can talk and hear and understand words as they travel in the air and come through my wired phone, much less a cellular phone!

But the day will come, and probably is here now, when we will communicate through only thought. We are still under the illusion that our thoughts are secret, not realizing that they, too, create in the visible world.

The ancient Chinese philosophy teaches that we live in an "energy field" and *our physical being is the result of the frequency of that field.* It also declares that every living species has its own unique energy frequency, differing from all the rest. As energy flows in a specific pattern, a specific visible formation will appear. We understand this as MRI's and EKG's and EEG's, as well as many other accepted tools of diagnostic study.

All things remain intact by this unseen energy, flowing in harmony, in perfect rhythm, *containing within itself the Eternal Order and Intelligence to maintain and sustain whatever it has formed physically.*

Plants have certain energy frequencies. Animals have their own specific energy frequencies. Planets, stars, suns all have yet another definite frequency of energy. It is out from these energies that these visible formations have developed.

To the casual observer it looks like a seed produced the new plant, a fertilized egg produced the new fish, bird, or human. But to examine deeper we find these seeds and eggs to be inanimate objects without the presence of the flow of this "energy of all Life."

Just as it is impossible for a sprout, as delicate and fragile as it is, in and of itself, to break open the confines of a shell, so is it impossible for a new galaxy of stars to burst forth from a sun except for the presence of the flow and activity of this energy of Life. Its Intelligence and Wisdom are unexplainable to the limited understanding of those who interpret life only from that which is seen.

To think that all visible life could have appeared of its own ability and then would be able to maintain and sustain itself, is to miss the real truth here. And that is that *Life is formed, maneuvered, animated, and directed by the invisible world of energy, which is the true substance of all form. We call this Presence LIFE. We call this flow and rhythm, this Intelligence and Wisdom, the Spirit of Life.*

Just as there are many branches on one tree, this One invisible Presence of Life has many and varied formations, many individual expressions of itself...and yet only one Life is the source of them all.

This is the Life of you and me.

It is in the understanding of this one Life, of its nature and varied characteristics, that we are finally able to understand ourselves, our thoughts and our bodies. It will be in this unfolding revelation that we will discover that our true existence, our true experience, is to be one of wholeness and goodness. Only then will we with any certainty and confidence reject the popular notion and acceptance of human misery and defeat, disease and decay.

So we are made in the *image* of God. The imagination, the thought of Divine Mind. All thought carries its own specific energy frequencies. Out from whatever thought is contained in the eternal Mind, out from its own nature, characteristics and specific attributes, we...as well as all creation...are formed. As we come forth from one eternal Mind and Being, we find that we are all visible formations made from the same source...*and that source is the substance of us all!* So we read in the first chapter of John, "Of His fullness have we all received."[1]

Now enters the theories, doctrines and beliefs of human kind...the human consciousness in direct contrast with the Divine Consciousness: humans trying to understand and define Life instead of allowing Life to define itself to us.

Science tells us that we are formed from specific DNA, genetic soup...the random formation of two individual sets of chromosomes.

This idea, while proven to the satisfaction of the minds of men, steeped in the consciousness of solid, physical matter as both cause and effect...leaves us the product of random activity of equally random energy. This is what I have come to call the law of chance and probability. If we agree to this ideology, we have every reason to live in fear and dread. Who knows then what hand we will be dealt. Life then becomes a game of poker...the best hand wins, the worst hand loses.

According to this philosophy, our personalities are already predetermined. Nothing we can do about it. My temperament, my likes and dislikes, my wants and demands, all are preordained, preprogrammed. No sense of personal responsibility or accountability in that fatalist ideology!

Following this line of reasoning, we will get whatever diseases we are programmed to get, so why are we bothering to try to escape? Why fight it? If it's in the genes, no matter how much we resist it, no matter how many vitamins we take, how many laps we do around the football field, no matter how many visits we make to the doctor's office, no matter how many diagnostic tests are ordered, we are going to get what we are going to get! Once again, this is living under the law of chance and probability.

However, if we subscribe to the belief that we all come from the same source, formed and created out from perfection, goodness, harmony and order; that we are governed by that which is the true substance of our being (not flesh and blood, but the Life energy of the Eternal One) and that this appearing is preordained unto goodness...we will soon realize a dramatic change in every aspect of our lives.

This is called living out from Truth and expecting that the truth, itself, will appear *defining its own nature.*

What science has done, by contrast, is examine what it *sees,* and then create an explanation to fit that which is already believed. We're getting what we are seeing and we're seeing what we are believing and we're believing what we have been told.

For instance, the human consciousness sees disease, suffering, deformity, sadness, death and disaster as its usual lot in life. We see this all around and about us and now need to find a reasonable cause for it all. But since we believe in physical causation, we look for the cause to appear in some physical form. The more we look in one direction, the more we are convinced of the reality of what we see.

But if we start with perfection and wholeness, uninterrupted goodness as the source of all life, we will bring that into our experience as surely as we have brought disaster.

We, by our thoughts and convictions, influence the flow of the energy field around and about us, and therefore, what we experience. We can understand and agree with the eternal flow of infinite energy (Spirit) or we can misunderstand and scramble the energy flow, leaving the field wide open for whatever to appear.

CHAPTER TWELVE

HEALTH VS. DIS-EASE

Now SIMPLY PUT, health is not merely the absence of symptoms in the physical or mental body...it is what we realize when this *Spirit of Life is easily and quietly flowing* through our minds, our attitudes, thoughts and emotions and through our bodies.

It brings with it clarity and purity of thought.

It brings gentleness and goodness in our desires and motives because its nature is Love.

It brings strength and energy and a sense of vitality.

It brings purpose and motivation and direction to our thought and to every cell and function of the body.

It brings order, balance and harmony.

This is what health should look and feel like to us.

Dis-ease on the other hand, is any place or space where that flow or presence of this Spirit of Life is blocked, congested, absent or simply not realized.

To release the congestion, to reestablish the flow of this Life is to realize health and strength once more.

It's all in the energy!

If we can grasp this, we can see how foolish and futile has been man's present effort of chasing disease with pills and more pills. It becomes increasingly apparent that to name, classify and categorize physical appearances of symptoms, along with endless chattering about various disease appearances, is mere madness. A declaration of a total lack of perception of Life. An evidence of living from an atmosphere of thought totally oblivious to the effect of one's thoughts and beliefs. Because the more we think and speak about this aberrant appearance called disease, the longer we allow it full rein within our imaginations, the greater the energy we give it and the greater its appearance.

This endless, mindless thought (and strength robbing effect) of such hysterical confusion, only serves to increase the congestion of the needed flow of this Spirit of Life, further propagating the evidences of disease.

There is a way to live free from the tyranny of disease, to live in a state of peace and quietness, where there is no dread or fear of sudden destruction or insidious deterioration of aging.

But rather than find it in a pill, or in the expertise of the wisdom and genius of a mere mortal man, we will discover it ourselves as we are quietly lifted into that place of understanding and as we yield to a complete and radical change in our perception of life. Finally allowing Life to define itself to us.

And as we are led into this new understanding and experience, we will discover that all we have sought to find, all we have frantically and elusively sought after, is already here.

CHAPTER THIRTEEN

WHAT IS THIS THING CALLED DISEASE?

DISEASE IS AN INTERRUPTION in the normal function of anything in life.

It is an interruption in the normal rhythm of life...of the normal integrity of life.

Dis-ease is an interruption in the "ease" or peaceful existence of any aspect of life.

The most important correction of thought needs to be that *disease is not a power* in and of itself, and it is not *something that appears*...but an ABSENSE of something. An absence of the flow of life...a glitch in an otherwise free flowing, life giving and life sustaining energy. Scrambled energy producing confusion, chaos, and disorder.

Disease is a nothing, a vacuum...a space formed when the presence of Life is not realized! Into which we create horrible images of thought, only originating from fear, mis-understanding and a sense of vulnerability.

The more we talk about it and the more we describe it in detail for the imagination of men to feed upon, the more real to our minds it becomes. Like a shadow in the dark until the light shines and the shadow disappears. A shadow can be anything our imagination will create until the fullness of light appears... and then it becomes nothing. When the fullness of understanding comes, you will also see that disease is nothing.

We must stop seeing it as *something...but only as the absence of something. An absence of the sense of the presence of Life.*

We must stop calling it by names and categories. We must stop identifying it according to where or how it appears. In this we are exalting it, honoring it. Building a shrine to it.

We must realize it is not many different diseases, varied and distinctive ...as varied and distinctive as the many millions of names we have graced it with. But it is just one common experience with many varied manifestations...*an experience of disorder.* An experience of confusion, chaos. An interruption in the flow of the current of life energy as it freely moves throughout all creation...forming, animating, motivating, sustaining, all that we see in this visible world.

It becomes critical to our understanding here that we begin to realize that Life is not what we are doing or experiencing from birth to death, as is humanly described...*it is a viable, real entity*...a Presence, a power, a force, an energy that *fills all space and place* and is not confined by anything made. *Indeed it made all that is made.*

Life then is another word for God.

The Spirit of Life is that portion of the Being of God that formed all things, and causes all things to exist in harmony, balance and perpetual order throughout all eternity.

It is as the air we breathe. It *is* the air we breathe. The Latin root prefix for the word air is *pneumo.* The same root prefix for the words, breath and spirit. Air, breath and spirit are all one...the Omnipresent Source of that which creates all and gives existence to all.

This Spirit of Life is intelligence and wisdom. It is order and harmony and beauty and perfection. Whereever it freely flows there is the evidence of intelligence, wisdom, harmony, order, beauty and perfection.

So what is disease?

It would have to be a place or space where the flow of Life is interrupted, or believed to be. A place where the energy is scrambled, blocked or restricted. Then what would appear would be something other than beauty, order and perfection. What would then appear would be anomalous, distorted, ugly and dark. Dis-ease. Otherwise known as confusion.

So then, no matter what appears, how it manifests, where it manifests...whatever names have been given it; no matter under what classification it appears...it is all simply a space or place of congestion where Life is not flowing!

If we picture this flow through our bodies as a river and realize the pure, clear appearance of the water when the river is freely flowing. We recognize that it is in this clear life giving water that fish and other water creatures can live.

We get the feeling of health and vibrant energy. We then turn our attention to areas where the water is trapped, stagnant...such as a lagoon or an eddy. It is in these places where fermentation appears. This is a breeding ground for every imaginable insect and creature. This is known as a swamp...murky and thick with crud and decay. This is disease.

In the Old Testament, the prophet, Ezekiel describes a "river of Life" that heals whatever it touches as it flows through human thought. This river of life proceeds out from the mind of God. It is the knowledge of that which is true and eternal. "Whatsoever it touches, is healed."[1]

But it warns against areas of swamp where the river does not flow. Those areas remain in a state of stagnation and decay.

The prerequisite to coming into this river of Life is to completely submerge yourself..."not to the ankles, not to the knees, not to the hips, but into the water so deep that you cannot pass over...but must be carried along by the flow of its current."[2]

This is surrender to the Mind of God, where we cease our own thoughts, schemes, worries and solutions. This is where we allow a higher consciousness, the knowledge of what is true, to fill in that space in our mind where only confusion ruled before. "And all things will become new."[3]

Immediately we realize the foolishness of trying to clear away the decay and death. We understand that even if we could succeed in clearing it all away, so long as the water is congested, it will only reappear. We know that a good rainfall will solve the problem. Just *get the river flowing.* To the degree that this area is opened up...it will then appear as the rest of the river. The health of the waters will reappear.

And so it is throughout all the varied manifestations of Life. Every formation of Life *needs the free flowing energy of the Spirit of Life in order for wholeness and vitality to be sustained.*

We must guard against any blockage or narrowing in the easy flow of Life *and we do this by watching our thoughts,* our beliefs. For it is not so much what we do or do not do that affects this river of Life through us, *as what we think* and believe.

One of the most insidious, prevailing contributions to disease in the whole of the collective human thought system is our belief about disease itself. We are like the guy trying to clean up the swamp, thinking that if we study every creature that breeds there we can somehow overcome it. Two hundred years of this kind of medical management with the swamp still happily breeding new and more horrific creatures every year ought to teach us that this is not the way of wisdom.

To date we are consumed by the presence of disease.

Fascinated by its terrible horrors.

Overwhelmed by its all pervasiveness.

It appears to have the capacity to change, alter, redirect, destroy and govern our lives, our thoughts, our resources.

We exercise extreme efforts to avoid it, while all the while *acknowledging its power over us.*

We fear its effects. We obey its demands.

We give it all the time, effort and energy it requires.

We talk about it incessantly.

Probably half of the inhabitants of the world are somehow connected to it, spending their lives either attempting to treat it, analyze it, annihilate it, chase it around with pills or other equally futile means, discovering new and innovative ways to examine it, building buildings that we can name after it.

It governs us.

It demands our respect, our thought, our fear, our substance.

It has become a god to us, in and of itself, and we have unknowingly built shrines to it.

While we collectively hate it...we are serving it. We cower and cringe in its presence...like a terrible king, a monster ruling authority, a brutal dictator.

We have erected great and magnificent edifices to it, like the slaves of the Egyptian Pharaohs, we writhe under the whip and torture it inflicts while we continue to build its pyramids, its cities, its castles...the great pharmaceutical companies, the towering medical complexes. We bow in fear and awe at its many images and its power to destroy.

We have honored it with great and swelling names, too difficult to properly pronounce...which only serves to make it even more awe inspiring.

We have analyzed, bisected, and dissected it till we have become walking, talking medical dictionaries, very proud of our knowledge and industry...and totally unaware that with all that knowledge we are digging our own graves.

I wonder when it will dawn upon us that disease is an illegitimate experience...with no intrinsic power of its own, no creator, no life of its own, no substance.

That instead of actually being something...*it is the absence of something only.*

Like a roaring lion with no teeth, no claws, it derives the only power that it has from what we in our fear, ignorance and idolatry have given it.

I wonder when it will dawn upon us that this, too, is another god that we have created in fear and ignorance of the truth...unto our own destruction.

CHAPTER FOURTEEN

DISSECTING DISEASE

First we declare that disease is a part of the human condition that is unavoidable. Next we declare that it is all powerful, more powerful than the body's resistance to it.

As a matter of fact, we are so entrenched in the various ramifications of disease that we have forgotten about the body's natural defenses against foreign invasion and degeneration.

When was the last time we heard about the wonders of the human body? When were we taught about the unsearchable wonders of its intelligence? When did we last hear anyone admit that we have not scratched the surface of understanding about it all?

Several years ago I found myself surrounded by patients who were suffering from leukemia. Diseases seem to come in waves. One patient in particular seemed to catch my attention more than the others. He was a cop from Houston, married with two small children.

One night I had a horrible dream about leukemia and for hours the next day I couldn't shake it. One of my patients noticed that I was out of sorts and asked me what was bothering me. She was a really neat Christian lady who carried a lot of wisdom, so I told her about my patients and this man in particular...and about my dream. She told me that I ought to be listening for wisdom from God about this situation. She felt that was why I had the dream, perhaps to stop fretting about the patients and begin to listen for the voice of wisdom. I knew when she spoke that she was right and immediately I began to 'expect' to hear something. I knew that I would.

Well, two days went by and not a word from God, but I wasn't discouraged. I knew I would hear something, I could feel it.

And finally on the third day I was reading a magazine that came to the house once a month that was spiritually inspiring with its articles and stories. I came across a short article written by a physician called, "Our Wondrous Body."[1]

He began talking about how *each specific aspect of the body declared the nature of Christ* and began to talk about the leukocytes! Wow! The hair on my arms stood up straight! Leukocytes are the immature white blood cells, waiting in the shadows of the bone marrow till they become mature enough to enter the blood stream as lymphocytes.

I knew this was what I had been waiting to hear. Leukemia is a disease concerning these young, immature white blood cells. No coincidence here!

He personalized a leukocyte, called him Luke, and began to share a day in the life of one baby white blood cell.

Luke, he wrote, was restless and anxious, wanting to get on with his purpose in life and join the other white blood cells in the blood stream. He wanted to fight infection and inflammation like the "big boys" got to. Day after day he waited until one day he got the message from an "M" cell that it was time for him to go. He was beside himself with excitement and dove into the blood.

Up the venous system he traveled and into the right atrium of the heart. Through the tricuspid valve and into the right ventricle, up the pulmonary artery and into the lungs. He was having the time of his life!

He knew what lay ahead of him would be a difficult battle, and would no doubt cost him his life, but he also knew that this was the reason for him to exist...to gladly give his life so that the whole of the body could live! Without one self serving thought in his heart, without a hint of self preservation, he swam on.

Back into the heart, now through the left atrium, bicuspid valve, left ventricle, out the aorta and down, down, down into the right iliac artery. His senses were attuned to the signals that outlined his course. Down the femoral artery to the foot.

Now things were getting difficult. The large toe was to be his destination, but the tissue swelling was so great that his way through the vascular system was impaired. So determined *to give his life that the whole may live*, he took on an amoeba-like form and oozed through the capillary wall into the tissue. Here the battle was intense. He could feel the heat. He could see his fellow white blood cells falling in battle even as they formed a circle to "wall off" the infection in the toe. Without hesitation he joined in the battle and through it all, he gave up his short life.

The result was the healing of the whole organism!

As the author was making the obvious comparison to the life and willing death of Jesus Christ to "save the whole," I was crying so hard I could almost not read the words.

All my "medical" life I was taught that the leukocytes were the "enemy" in leukemia. They were believed to be the cause of the disease...never once were they depicted as being in such numbers and force to "protect" the body. Instead they were targeted for chemotherapy until they died!

All of a sudden I was "in love" with those little guys. I wanted to protect them from what was being done to them. I wanted them to know that I understood why they came out in such numbers...not to hurt, but to help an already over-toxic body, to deal with the very toxins that would destroy it.

So, as stupid as this probably sounds, I stretched across my bed and thanked them for their constant sacrifice and for their willingness to unflinchingly forfeit their life for the life of the whole.

I really fell in love with the body as a whole that day, realizing that every cell, organ and structure did exactly the same thing all day, everyday. There was not one self-serving, self-preserving thought contained within the entire function of the body.

The body, then, was as the whole of creation, a visible expression of the love of God. The willing sacrifice of love. And here we were, in our blind, arrogant ignorance... misunderstanding it, resisting it, and destroying it!

The last time I had seen this man was just three days prior to this experience. At that time his "white count" was roaring at over one hundred thousand! The next time I saw him was the following week, three days after my new understanding and his white count was down to a normal 7,000! To my knowledge it never again raised outside the parameters of normal.

With that experience I gained a respect for our bodies that was lost in all the study of disease. I gained an awareness of the Divine intelligence of it. I realized the life of it was really the eternal Life of God.

I experienced a complete shift in perception whereby *the disease became fragile and the body strong.* This was a huge shift.

The entire world has been "educated" in the power of disease and the frailty of the human body to resist it, thereby needing the myriads of drugs and medical interventions.

I began to realize that the *whole of creation,* not just the body, was a visible demonstration of the nature of God...*if only we had eyes to see that and a heart to understand.* Thus the omnipresence of God.

There are three scriptures that come to mind here that declare to me the all-ness of God...which precludes the appearance of anything unlike His nature...such as disease:

Psalms 19: 1-3. "The heavens declare the glory of God, and the firmament shows his handiwork. Day unto day utters speech (everything that appears each day is teaching us the nature of God) and night unto night shows us knowledge. There is no speech nor language where their voice is not heard. (All over the world creation declares the message) Their words are gone out through all the earth, even to the end of the world."

Romans 2: 20. "For the invisible things of God (nature, attributes) from the creation of the world, are clearly seen, being understood by the things which are made."

Job 12: 7, 8. "But ask now the beasts of the field, and they shall teach thee. And the fowls of the air, and they shall tell thee. Or speak to the earth and it shall teach thee, and the fishes of the sea shall declare it unto thee."

Job might just as well have said, "Ask now your body and it will tell you and teach you of the glory of God. Ask your cells and ask your bone marrow. Ask the immune system and the variety of white blood cells. Ask the endocrine (hormonal balancing system) and it will declare the nature of the infinite God to you."

We have a choice here. We chose to fear our body, to criticize it and find continual fault with it. We chose to not trust it at all. By doing so we chose to not trust its Maker.

We read again and again that Christ (the visible expression of the invisible God) is manifest in our body. That the wisdom and person of God fills all that it has formed. That God is not separate from the thing which he has created...including our body.[2] But we have listened to the "wisdom" of man, which has turned out to be the fear and ignorance of man, and have been swept away by the words. From this collective human consciousness we must escape!

SECTION TWO

INTRODUCTION

In this section we are going to travel down a path of a new and fresh introduction into the nature of God and how this understanding completely changes our relationship to God as the source and origin of all existence.

We will discover how a shift in understanding about God will cause us to see life from a different perspective. We will begin to realize ourselves in a different light and find that this will, in turn, produce different results in our life experiences.

Most of all we will have the boldness to find entrance into the heart and Mind of God. There we will see as He sees, know as He knows and live as He sent us to live. This is the only way, and the only hope, for us to live in peace... within our bodies, our minds and our world.

CHAPTER ONE

RETHINKING OLD CONCEPTS

"It is given unto you to know the
mysteries of the kingdom of God"[1]

To EMBARK UPON THE FORMIDABLE TASK of re-introducing you to God is indeed an ambitious undertaking, but that is exactly what I am going to attempt to do. For me, learning a new and more pure understanding of God has made all the difference in the world in my life and in the lives of those who have come to me for help throughout the years.

My understanding of the nature and person of God, compared to what had been formed in my mind throughout the years previously, is as the proverbial day and night. I now *expect* goodness to prevail in my life, where before I looked only for conflict. I find that peace and serenity is God's *natural order* of the day, instead of accepting the notion that conflict and confusion are the tools employed by God to correct the error of human activity. Whereas previously I found only turmoil in an acute sense of overwhelming responsibility to "make life work," I now enjoy the immutable truth that Life is always working in perpetual Divine order. I only needed to allow it to appear as such in my heart to see the truth of that.

I finally came to realize that I no longer needed to agree to pain and defeat to atone for my 'miserable existence' (although I had no idea that I was doing that) and instead, I could allow myself the luxury of expecting and living in a perpetual atmosphere of acceptance and goodness.

But the most startling change was that *my opinion of myself and everyone else changed as my understanding of God was restructured*. Now I was able to see creation through the heart of God and to know the eternal and present beauty and glory of it all.

Once again I need to refer to the scripture in the Old Testament in the book of II Samuel, chapter 22, which says, "With the merciful thou will show thyself merciful, and with the upright man thou will show thyself upright. With the pure thou will show thyself pure. But with the judgmental and hardness of men's hearts, thou will show thyself unyielding." Did God appear differently to different folks? And was that because we saw only what we *could* see based upon our present understanding? And how much of that understanding was formed by what we had learned of God through the creed and dogma of man? I knew I needed to know God as God truly is and no longer simply be carried along by the prevailing ignorance into further destruction.

One of the most difficult perception shifts to take place for me was the idea that *we* could change, direct, or otherwise have anything to do with the events that took place in our lives. I was used to praying and asking a remote God to change, direct or otherwise correct things that happened to me or those who came for prayer. Sometimes those prayers were answered and sometimes not.

Now I was beginning to realize that *we were experiencing life according to our understanding* and it was that very understanding that needed to be corrected. In other words, my focus needed to change from asking God to correct *the effect of what we believed*, to correcting what was being believed in the first place.

Soon my prayers changed and instead of focusing on improving human conditions, I began to desire to know truth, to know what was contained in the Eternal Wisdom and knowledge of God on any particular subject. As that began to be revealed to me, the desired change in the human condition automatically appeared.

Even so, I wasn't sure that I liked the idea of being placed in the position of being responsible for thinking and knowing "right" so that "right" would appear. It seemed so much safer to simply rely on whatever was "the will of God" for any particular situation and then just "coast" my way through. I found that I was afraid of what I erroneously perceived as a personal responsibility to bring forth this new understanding, this higher atmosphere of thought. But something happened one day at the clinic that made me see how simple and sure this new way of prayer would be for me.

❧

Midmorning one day I received a frantic call from a very close friend of mine. She was at the hospital with her husband who had become suddenly and critically ill several days before with what was diagnosed as acute ulcerative colitis. This caused aggressive colon hemorrhaging, continual diarrhea and rapid weight loss. He had already dropped 30 to 35 pounds in a very short time and was now weak and severely anemic. The only treatment that was being offered was to remove the large colon. She was calling for prayer because she was just informed that in one hour that was what was going to happen!

My head began to whirl in response to her anxiety. I found myself vacillating between the old traditional concept of God Who must be appealed to and then may or may not respond...and my new understanding of the present perfection of man in His image, regardless of what may appear to challenge this.

I immediately excused myself from the patient I was working with and went out to sit in my car so I could be quiet for a minute. I asked God, "How should I pray?" I heard the answer before I finished asking the question. *"Pray to see that only the Mind of God is prevailing."* So I did. I included the patient, his wife, myself, the doctors and hospital staff and anyone else who was aware of his problem. I reasoned that God was the intelligence and government of all that He formed in His image and out from His likeness. That being the eternal truth, all those involved would naturally be in one accord and would be under the wise counsel of Divine Mind.

It occurred to me that *every single challenge to mankind, every problem, every untoward event is really a challenge to this very truth.*

In every problem that man faces, the present belief is that something other than the eternal goodness of God is governing the situation. To declare and really *know* that God, who is omnipresent and omnipotent, is always and continually governing in Divine Order and perfection is the solution for each problem that arises.

In five minutes I was back inside taking care of business at the clinic.

An hour later she called me to say that his last blood work had remained constant, so they had decided to wait for a couple of hours to see what would happen. Soon she reported to me that the second blood work was improving, so the surgery was indefinitely postponed. That night I went to the hospital to support them and we prayed and rejoiced in the "all ness" of God, who is only good and the "nothingness" of the horror of evil...refusing to give it the power that belonged only to God.

In just days he was home, all bleeding and convulsive colon disorder had stopped. He gained his weight back in just weeks and never to this day, over twenty years later, did this ever reappear.

Clearly this was a sure indication to me of the simplicity of what I was learning, as well as the truth of it. "To *know* Him truly is life eternal,"[2] Right here and now!

As I began to understand that *human life improves as our vision of God improves*, I was on a mission to pursue this at any cost.

It didn't take long to realize that everywhere I went for

understanding only led to further confusion. Men seemed to complicate even the most reasonable of thoughts. Religion was fraught with fears and contradictions. So I turned to the only sensible source available, and that was God, Himself. "You have no need that any man should teach you, but the anointing which lives within, will lead and guide you into all truth."[3]

I thought about this continually and found great comfort and strength in my hours and days asking various questions of the Spirit of Truth[4] and allowing the answers to be formulated in my mind and heart. This has taken all the years of my life, to undo and redo my image of Who and what God is, what the nature and characteristics are, and what my relationship and responsibilities are to it. But it has been such a wonderful experience and one that I wouldn't trade for anything or anyone.

I found the answers and 'unfolding understandings' to be quite sure and exact, often accompanied with astonishing events of healings of those that I had been caring for. At each turn God was there to seal the understanding with unprecedented proofs and surety. It became my personal goal in my life, far surpassing any other which appeared along the way, and the reward for the diligence has been beyond that which I ever expected or sought.

Plain and simple, God has a nature with definite characteristics, just as everything created and formed does. To know these is to know God. To know these is to know ourselves as well, for we are made in the exact image of His nature.

This is where we have a tendency to lose it, because *we*

judge by what we see and unfortunately we see only what we have been taught to see. We must learn to "judge righteously."[5] That is to judge as God sees, not as man sees.

This being the undeniable case, we must realize that to re-know something, we will around every corner find ourselves challenged by what we have learned. This often produces conflict and struggle within. While the Spirit of Truth reveals the pure understanding, the old imagery fights to hold on. I have found that things go much smoother, and the results are much more able to be received as pure truth, if I stay as far out of the struggle as possible. I could certainly feel the tension within, but I learned to resist believing that it was my responsibility to jump in with my reasonings and opinions and arguments. Even so, early on I would often find myself arguing against the new thought as it was attempting to appear, even though admittedly the old belief was never clear to start with. But all that soon subsided as I grew in understanding and trust of the process.

I started out 'knowing that I didn't know.' That was a prerequisite to learning... *being humble enough to know that I really didn't know anything at all.* So what would convince me to enter my opinions now that the Truth was revealing itself to me? I found that it all gets sorted out soon enough if I just stay quiet and still, don't discuss the thoughts and ideas with anyone as they roar around inside my heart... and wait. Without my erroneous and feeble input, the truth, the pure understanding, will always prevail.

I also found that I was often afraid to "let go" of something that I had been taught to believe, for fear that by letting go I would be bringing upon myself some sure destruction from God. But soon I realized that that unnatural fear of punishment from God was just the very thing that He was removing from my heart as I learned more of His calm, quiet, immutable and gentle nature and His undeniable desire that I know Him as He truly is.

I reasoned that if I came to Him for truth and understanding of Him, He would direct my learning, what I read, who I came in contact with, what I was hearing, etc. And, like our kidneys which He created to remove unnecessary substances from the body, He would also allow to pass from my *thinking* anything which was not going to be of any benefit to remain.

In short I learned to trust and to completely depend upon Him, the Spirit of Truth, to lead me and guide me from understanding to understanding until I came face to face with Him as He really is. And how different that turned out to be! How life-giving and what peace prevailed!

The question might arise at this point as to why this is so important to us. How exactly does this information play out in our lives? Is it able to help our immediate concerns? Heal our diseases? Repair our marriages? Bring our sons and daughters back home? Meet our financial needs?

And the answers to all these questions and more is that there *is a direct link, a connection between our image of God and what we allow into our lives and into our experiences.*

❧

If I believe, for instance, that God punishes us for our

many offenses by sending or allowing disease to appear on our bodies… then what is to be gained by asking Him to heal me? At what point is His "anger" finally appeased?

But if I know that *"He does not reward me according to my iniquity,"*[6] then I will reject the notion that this pain and suffering is from God and I will be much more confident of receiving my healing.

Then to take this thought even further, if I come to *know* that I am made in the image of God, and that I am in a state of perpetual Divine Order, an object of Love itself, a child of Light… that enables me to *really feel* continual, perpetual order and uninterrupted perfection, then there would be no room for disease to appear in my experience in the first place, would there? And if it tried, and I found myself challenged by disease, I would have the strength, confidence, power and truth to send it away. And it would leave.

"Whatsoever God hath made, it shall be forever, nothing can be added to it, nor anything taken from it." It would be upon that basis that I would live disease free and free of the fear of disease.

Do you see, just in that one example, how critical it is for us to know the true and pure understanding of not only God, *but us in His image and likeness as well*? There will never be a more important study in your life. There will never be a more challenging study in your life. And there will never be a more rewarding study in your life. Of all the things that man can devise to give his life to, this is without a doubt the most fulfilling. This is the next, best wilderness to be explored.

CHAPTER TWO

MY PERSONAL TRANSITION

MANKIND HAS BEEN SEARCHING for the true identity of God, its Creator, ever since the beginning of time. Religious historians and Biblical and social scholars have documented the various revelations from God to man on the subject of His nature and character and have found that it has been a progressive journey of understandings as we have been able to grasp it.

It is not that the truth changes. It *is* the truth of God and our origin, and therefore has not, nor could it ever change. It is only that our ability to comprehend such incomprehensible knowledge must be revealed slowly so that we can change our ideas and beliefs at a pace tolerable to us. Making this transition of thought was particularly gut wrenching for me.

For years I prayed and asked God why some people never seemed to get sick and others never seemed to have a moment of health. Why are some able to rise up and above a potential devastating experience and others appear trampled from the start?

While the world applauded science newest and greatest discovery, "genetic codes," to determine not only events that would happen in our lives, but how we would face them... I really ached for the truth. I found the general lack of the need to challenge these "discoveries" alarming and the attitude of the masses apathetic.

1984 was the beginning of one of the most devastating times in my personal life. The darkness was beyond description, known only to those who have also found themselves in such a condition. The end of this siege however, found me finally deeply convinced of the absolute truth of all that I had begun to understand. All confusion and the vacillating between the old concepts and the new were gone. I was finally ready to embrace this truth with all of my heart and soul.

I was daily managing the clinic with only one employee (we now have about 20). I was a "one man band" and we were seeing about 35 plus patients a day! I was devoutly raising my two daughters, pastoring a small group of about 75-100, and my home was full of folks from a church group in Alaska, all of them surrounding and supporting a young woman who was diagnosed with breast cancer.

In the meantime my children and I were adjusting to the first honest-to-goodness love relationship that I had allowed into our lives since their father left us 10 years before. This impossible full-plate began in 1980.

In 1984 the young woman passed away, two dear

patients who had survived cancer and heart disease were killed in car accidents, the "church group" dissolved, all 18 people moved out of my home, and my one brave try for a serious relationship crumbled.

At least the clinic remained standing and thriving. My heart was shattered, but worse than that I was so terribly disappointed and confused about God. You see, I prayed every prayer imaginable for this young woman, who died leaving behind three tiny children and hundreds of people stunned in disbelief. (She was the wife of a prominent preacher and was being "prayed for" by hundreds of folks who knew and loved them). As I said, I prayed (sometimes all night long), I fasted, I read and memorized every related scripture, believing without a doubt that she would recover. I left no "back door" of emotional support, just in case she didn't.

But the worst for me came during her memorial service, which was attended by several hundred confused and questioning souls, and a handful of preachers who claimed to have their answers. I finally came to the pinnacle of my search for truth. I was forced to let go of the last bare threads of traditional religion with all of its convoluted traditions of thought and endless processions of words. One by one the ministers spoke. Their pathetic groping for answers was obvious (as had been mine for the past ten years).

One declared that this woman's death was the "will of God," while the next loudly gave the devil all the credit. Back and forth they went. The dichotomy of thought, the emptiness of true understanding, wasn't missed by a single soul in that auditorium.

When it was my turn to speak, I simply confessed, with

tears of grief and frustration rolling down my face, that I had no idea anymore what to think or what to know. To blame God for the unprecedented horror that she endured was to have an image of God harder than the heart of Stalin or Hitler. To blame a devil was to deny the ability of God to correct, to deliver, to hear our prayers, to care. It was to have evil more powerful than God (good).

I announced that I was going back to San Antonio (the service was in Georgia) and wait...no matter if it took the rest of my life...until I knew whatever it was that I obviously didn't know about God. I meant it and they knew it!

Suddenly hundreds of people flew to their feet and clapped and cried with me. I knew then that hearts all over the world were aching to know more. It wasn't just roaring in my own soul, but all over people had come to the end of one era of understanding and were more than ready for the next truths to be revealed. The Bible calls that experience, leaving behind the old "landmarks" to expand and embrace new understandings. I call it leaving "one atmosphere of thought" and entering another. Some folks will never do it. Others won't be able to resist, for their hearts are aching and will not be silenced.

I am reminded of a scripture in the Old Testament Levitical law, one of many given to Moses to govern the children of Israel, until the true self-government appeared within their own hearts as the Christ.[1]

Here the children of Israel were instructed not to build houses or any permanent structure as they traveled through their wilderness experience toward the Promised Land. (The

Promised Land is speaking of the fullness of truth and understanding of the knowledge of God which creates heaven here in our earth experience..."Thy will be done on earth as it is in heaven."] Instead they were to live in tents only.

The obvious understanding here is that to "build a house" is to reside in a particular "atmosphere of thought" permanently, never desiring or allowing anything new to enter thought. Those who heed this warning and are willing to stay open and receptive to the Spirit of Truth, moving with the cloud by day and the pillar of fire by night,[2] with its progressive revelations of God and man, will not allow themselves to remain in one arena of thought forever. Of course this takes courage and trust. One must determine early on that it will be through prayer and revelation that they will continue to progress, and not by blindly following "every wind of doctrine" that blows their way. The sheep who listen only for the Master's voice will surely recognize it when it speaks. And another they will not follow![3]

So for five years I wandered through the wilderness of "thought," feeling very alone and willing to remain so, until something would be revealed to me which would elevate my understanding and radically correct my entire perception of the nature of God... who we are and why we are, and what this is really all about.

CHAPTER THREE

DOCTRINE OF THE
NECESSITY FOR SUFFERING

I KEEP SAYING THAT DISEASE IS ILLEGITIMATE. It is a man made concept that has as its foundation a human self image of failure, defeat, self loathing (which oftentimes disguises itself as pride). Then when we as humans "act out or live out," from that image of ourselves, we are punished for it. This is the premise upon which all "religious" thought is birthed. And we go downhill from there.

Remember that there is a universe of distinction between Religion and Spirituality.

One comes from the thought and conclusions of man, and therefore is subject to changeableness and error. It comprises a system of laws designed to bring us to a state of acceptability to God and a measure of holiness, although never really believing we could ever fully attain that.

The other comes from the mind of God and is eternal and immutable (unchangeable).

It declares our true identity to be eternally intact, not something to be attained, but something to accept. It describes the relationship between God and man to be one of *uninterruptible oneness*, God being the very Life of man. It requires our steadfast belief in the face of sometimes overwhelming appearances to the contrary in order for it to appear.

One brings the joy and goodness of Life in God, the other the pains and anguish of suffering and death.

Religion teaches us to see ourselves as miserable wretched sinners who deserve suffering and indeed *need* suffering to ever "get right." It is this concept, this belief, this ideology of human thought that acts as a magnet, drawing to us the necessary situations which will ensure our suffering! We "act out" from this image of ourselves. Change the image and we will find that we have changed the human situation.

CHAPTER FOUR

DOES GOD REWARD AND PUNISH?

PRETTY MUCH THE ENTIRE COLLECTIVE HUMAN thought believes that we are constantly being judged by God and that we always somehow turn up a failure when judged according to His impossible-to-reach standard of righteousness.

It is true that as humans we live under a "law of cause and effect," also called the "law of sowing and reaping." This comes from the verse in scripture that says, "Whatsoever you sow, that shall you also reap."[1] This is, of course, not referring to crops that come up from seeds sown in the earth. This is really referring to our thoughts, our words and our beliefs. Whatever we hold in thought as true is what we will "see" or experience.

Rather than realizing that *our image of God, of Life, is what is attracting pain and disease*, we are told and believe that it is God who has determined we should experience it. Indeed, this thought dominates throughout the entire history of man in his search for the understanding of life. This idea is well documented and unequivocally embraced by those who lived during the Old Testament writings, and lives on today in every traditional church in the land.

This confusion, calling God the progenitor of suffering, (always in response to our sinful nature) instead of realizing it is simply the fulfillment of a basic human law of sowing and reaping, is what has given us this erroneous concept of the nature of God. As it turns out, it is we, by our beliefs and actions, that draws to us our suffering.

It has also trapped us into believing we have no recourse except to beg God to remove what He has done, or begin the never ending exercise of trying in vain to overcome our sins and weaknesses. If we fail, we sink into an abyss of self condemnation. If we, by our standards of right behavior, succeed...we become self righteous, condemning all who, by this same standard, have failed.

I call this whole self effort, "climbing the mountain of morality." Just when you think you might be getting to the top another flaw in your character rises up to greet you and you know that there is no end to it all.

I spent years trying to be what the religious community wanted me to be. I watched every word I said and every response that surfaced in my soul. I was so intent on "appearing right" so that I could be a part of the "club." I, instead, became a nervous wreak and finally threw up my hands in utter exhaustion and quit trying altogether. The judgment was so extreme and my ability was so inferior...

Much to my amazement it was at that point that a warm and peaceful feeling swept over my heart and I began to know that I had been okay with God all along. He liked me just as I was, with all the rough edges and all the social flaws. It was that realization which led me to fall in love with God instead of serving him through fear. I felt accepted and loved. Any changes that took place in my life and in my person came through this change in consciousness, not because of any previous human effort. This time the changes stuck!

As we are locked into this error of thought we are unable to see that a *shift in understanding* is all that it will take for us to be free and clear of all attraction to pain and confusion.

When we read that we are to love our enemies, those who sin against us, do we think that God would do less than what He tells us to do? The words that follow "Love those who wrong you" are, "For God makes his sun to rise on both the evil and the good and sends rain on the just and the unjust alike."[2]

Now where is the judgment and punishment in that thought?

In the very Bible from which religion teaches we have *earned* this suffering, we read, "Blessed is the man who realizes that the Lord does not reward us according to our iniquity."[3]

GOD AS THE ONE LIFE OF ALL CREATION

We read in the first chapter of the Bible that man began with an image of himself as pure, perfect, whole, complete and beautiful. He was one with God, walked with God and felt loved and totally unafraid. He had no idea what fear was. He had no reason to know such a thing. (Whether you choose to read the story as actual fact or an allegory makes no difference here.)

He was told to always "eat of the tree of life." This means that he was to "see" life everywhere, feel its beauty and enjoy its goodness.

Again, life is not what we are doing as humans...*life is God*. From the beginning there was only *one Life* and out from that one Life all visible manifestations appeared. The Spirit of the One Life gave impulse to everything formed. "For from Him and through Him and to Him are all things."[1]

As long as this continued in our thought we gloried in the wonders of this Life.

At the same time we were cautioned never to judge anything as right or wrong, good or evil...for in the day we would do this we would die! This is what is meant by "eating of the tree of the knowledge of good and evil."[2]

Because to thus judge, you must first separate that which you are judging from the Life that is flowing through it and animating it. You must first believe that this part of creation is a separate entity from the One Life and so could fall into evil. You have just divided God...at least in your mind. We are never to judge "according to appearances,"[3] but instead to look beyond what appears to the never changing Life, which is the true substance of all things. This is called judging "righteous judgment," and that we *are* told to do!

We were instructed, and still are, to *see only Life* when viewing all things and all people. To see God *in and as* all things.

We must teach ourselves to see this Life, instead of the mortality of a person, or a thing created. This will keep us from judging them as "good or evil," "right or wrong," "healthy or sick." This will keep us from judging *ourselves* as "good or evil," "right or wrong."

This insisting on *seeing the true Life* of them will also *call it forth* into expression. This is how we are to love and heal one another.

The more we practice this, the less we engage in thoughts of "my life," or "your life," or "his or her life." Soon we will recognize that there really only is one Life and as we come to this understanding, the glory of that Life appears.

෬

Back to the Garden of Eden…

Now along comes the serpent.[4] The Hebrew word for 'serpent' means 'fear.' This entity of thought suggests that God is both good and evil, declaring that God is capable of withholding good from us whenever He sees fit to do so. The serpent suggested here that God was withholding wisdom and understanding from his beloved, man, thus impregnating the heart of man with the thought that he is separate and inferior.

As soon as man heard these words and believed them, he *ate* of the knowledge of both good and evil. This means that he partook of this lie. He thus began a life of judgment, and therefore a life of fear. He judged God as capable of both good and evil. He judged himself as capable of both good and evil. And he judged everything else as capable of both good and evil.

In the new-found judgment of man, he even began to "name" certain animals, as being either kind and gentle or capable of viciousness…harming, poisoning, being unpredictable and living by fear themselves.

Now man saw himself as naked. Naked means unclothed from the beauty and glory of the One Life. It means separate and isolated and alone. No longer does man see himself as a part of the One Life. Now he is afraid of the God that made him. He cannot trust the goodness of God anymore. He believes goodness, in any form, could be withheld.

He feels personally responsible for his own life now, no longer allowing the Spirit of the One Life to flow through him, manifesting the glory of God's Life.

So man sees himself as naked and is ashamed! The word ashamed here means "to lack." No longer does man see himself as possessing all things and always enjoying the abundant goodness of Life. Suddenly man believes he is lacking and therefore needing to secure goodness for himself. Now he is responsible for his life...he is on his own!

In shame and fear he hides behind a bush. What are the bushes in our life? Where do we run from our terrible feelings of unworthiness, isolation and fear? What do we do to "squash" these unbearable feelings? Do we pretend they are not there?

Our bush is whatever we engage in which successfully *distracts us* from the truth of God, and us, as an expression of His One life.

Alcohol? Prescription drugs? Soap operas? Endless talking on the telephone? Working or shopping till we drop? Preoccupation with our bodies? Multitudes of doctor visits? Preoccupation with entertainment, with sex, with the lives of people who are well known?

All this began when we believed that God was the author of both good and evil. He then became the judge of our goodness or our failures and therefore the one who rewarded or punished, whichever the case may be.

Instead of living the One Life and enjoying it, we began to live to *earn* goodness, but all the while *expecting* bad to happen.

In all this, God said to Adam and says today, "Who told you that you were naked? Who told you to be ashamed? Who told you I was the progenitor of good and evil? Who told you to be a judge of good and evil?"

The truth here is that if God were both good and evil, He would be a house divided and unable to stand. He would self destruct and taste of death Himself, since from his own mouth He declared that such a dichotomy of thought produced death. "In the day you know good and evil, you shall surely die."

If God judges our right and wrong, He must *see and know evil* and that makes Him eligible for death Himself. If God does not judge our right or wrong as we have all our lives been told, then what does He see and know about us?

What God knows is what He has made...not what we have made from our misunderstandings and fears. What God knows is what He is. There is only One Life and that Life is God and God means "good."

So God really only sees pure and perfect, whole and complete Life. He knows only harmony, order and balance in all things. He knows only goodness and joy and gladness. And all this is called the glory of God.

Once we know the truth, from our hearts, about God and about man, we discover that in every case *God is on our side*. We can now step out from behind whatever bush we have been hiding. We can feel ourselves fully clothed by Goodness and Love and Worthiness and Innocence. We can at this moment in time receive all the abundance of good that is God...that is our Life!

God is our beloved Creator, the source and origin of all life. In His eyes, it is impossible for any part of His creation to fall into damage or disrepair.

Looking now at what we all know to be the true nature and character of God, we realize how utterly impossible it is for God to be the progenitor of evil...for any reason. We can then understand how utterly illegitimate the whole experience of disease really is.

Disease is an "accepted" evil, an accepted violence. When we come to the place of understanding *why* we don't need to accept it anymore, we will then cease to experience it. The mass mesmerism, mass hypnotic hysteria will let go of its hold on our hearts and minds and we will be free. "Then the inhabitants of the land shall no more say, "'I am sick.'"[5]

CHAPTER SIX

GOD AS UNCHANGABLE GOODNESS

As my understanding of the nature of God grew I learned to stop calling Him God. That word alone brought up old pictures and beliefs keeping me from being able to learn anything new.

So instead I began to refer to God according to His Eternal Nature and not just the name, "God."

For instance, I learned that the word *God* came from the Saxon word for *good*. So I began to think of God as all goodness. For a long time I stayed with that. It reinforced to me that if God was all good, then it would not be consistent to expect bad to come from Him.

I found that the longer I stayed with that thought I could ask anything, leave it with God and trust that whatever the solution was, it could only be good. Before this understanding came I had this perpetual thought that God might send something bad to me, for my own good, of course! This made me afraid to trust God for good, so I lived my life separate and apart from the Wisdom and Counsel of God. I just tried to figure it all out for myself and do the best that I could. When I did begin to pray, I erroneously believed that I needed to *tell* God what needed to be done and how, because I didn't trust His goodness or His Wisdom.

Another mile marker came when I learned the word *immutable.* To realize that God was *unchangeable* goodness meant to me that He was *not reactive.* God did not bless me with good if I earned it, nor did God curse me with bad just because in my judgment of myself, I earned it. *God was constant in all His attributes and in all His nature.* Nothing I did or didn't do could change anything about the goodness of God.

Religion has God changing every time we do. It's unnerving and inconsistent. There is no secure foundation in that thought. "I am the Lord, thy God. I change not."[1]

It was true that my actions and most of all, my beliefs, still determined my experience, but if I only stopped and *"moved my thought into the truth of the presence of the goodness of God,"* all things changed for good. I found a way to *transcend the law of cause and effect!*

When I was in error, I simply had to realize that I was stuck in the human vision of life but now desired to be in the presence of only God's vision of life. With that desire came a whole new understanding and experience...always.

James declares, "He is the Father of lights (you and me) with whom is no variableness, neither shadow of turning."[2] This speaks of God as immutable, not reactive and unchanging.

Nothing we believe, do, or fail to do, will ever change what God has done, or what God sees and knows. *I can suffer from my false beliefs, but when I turn to the Spirit of Truth to show a better way I find unchangeable goodness...every time.* This refutes the theory that we serve a God of reward and punishment.

We serve a God of goodness. We only need to move from our present thought (belief) into the consciousness of the Mind and Truth of God.

CHAPTER SEVEN

GOD AS SPIRIT

UNFORTUNATELY, MOST OF US STILL SEE God as a man. We say that we don't, but we do. We judge the nature of God to be as the nature of a man. The whole Old Testament writings do that. We read that God is jealous, angry, requiring just retribution and demanding impossible sacrificing and suffering to cause Him to change His present course of action. We have Him sorry that He made certain choices and determined to correct His previous decisions.

The reason for these inconsistencies is that we speak what we understand. This was what men understood and their highest sense of truth was what they recorded.

You will notice how radically the images of truth changed when Jesus entered the scene. He brought a sense of God as Spirit, as attributes of a nature, more than a person. And yet he personalized God by calling Him, Father, the source of all being. He introduced God in a way that men could not perceive at that time and for the most part still don't.

He told us that in the kingdom of God there is neither male nor female. That makes God neither male nor female...but Life and Love, Itself.

When Paul began to teach, he further declared that *man, made in the image of this nature...was the manifestation of this nature in the earth. He called it the "mystery of godliness."*[1]

Later John, captured by the Love that is God, went so far as to describe the relationship between God and man by saying, "Herein is your love made perfect, that you should have the boldness to say, 'As He is in heaven, so are we in the earth.'"[2]

You can see how the Bible is a progressive unfolding of truth from God to man, correcting his understandings and causing him to appear as he was intended. But the understanding is there for us to have and to possess. "It is your Father's good pleasure to give you the kingdom,"[3] to give us depth of perception and clarity of thought.

We will appear as He is, but only when we *see* Him as He truly is. "And you shall be like him, when you see him as he is"[4]

CHAPTER EIGHT

THE KEY TO THE KINGDOM...
HOW TO SEE THE TRUTH

T HE FUNNY THING ABOUT God is that His ways are not our ways.

We think that perhaps to simply say the words, read the words, sing the words...we will somehow become the words.

But the way is clear: *to go up, you must first be willing to go down.*

There were once two men who came to where Jesus was staying and asked Phillip if they could see him. When Phillip told Jesus that these men desired to see him, he answered in this very mysterious way.

"Tell them that unless a kernel of wheat falls to the ground and dies, it abides alone, but if it dies it brings forth much fruit. Tell them that he who is willing to *lose his life, will gain it.* But he who clings to his life will lose it. Tell them that they need to take up their cross and follow me."[1] Then and only then could they ever really "see" him.

Jesus was humble enough to know that they were not nearly as interested in meeting him as in seeing was what it was *about* him that made him so different from other men. What caused him to be able to do the things he did and know the things he knew. He understood that they needed to see him *everywhere and in every person*. He perceived what they really needed to see was truth, and to know how to get to it.

So he told them how to see the unseen, do the undoable, and know the unknowable.

☙

Be willing to lose the present sense of your life. Cease to live for yourself. Be willing to let another sense of Life emerge. Begin to live to fulfill the purpose for which you have been sent. In other words, "take up this 'cross' daily and follow the way that I have taken."

The cross is the place where *one life is exchanged for another*. At least one "sense of life" is denied so that a new sense of life might emerge.

"Then you will see me! And when you see me you shall be like me."

☙

So Paul, with the message loud and clear wrote, "For to me to live is Christ, to die is gain."[2] And still in another place he said, "I die daily."[3] Meaning that he daily *chooses to choose*...that the life he once thought he lived was not that life which he was sent to live...therefore he "dies to one" that the other might be revealed.

We are referring to consciousness here and not actions or behavior. Religion wants us to exercise behavior. To act a certain way, think a certain way and believe a certain way. *But God wants a complete change in consciousness.*

Remember that the cross is the place where one sense of who we are is exchanged for another. It requires a *strong sense of purpose and deliberate decision...daily.*

CHAPTER NINE

HUMAN CONSCIOUSNESS VS. DIVINE CONSCIOUSNESS

WHILE THERE ARE MANY DISTINCT DIFFERENCES between the human consciousness and the Divine consciousness, there are two that we can discuss here. One is concerned with our focus and intention of life, the other is concerned with our interpretation of life.

The first law of the human is "Survival of the fittest. Do unto others before they do it unto you. Look out for number one first. Get out and get it! The early bird catches the worm! Might is right. God helps those who help themselves." (Now where in the earth did that one come from?)

By contrast, the first law of God is "Love is not love till there is a sacrifice involved. Give, with no thought for yourself. Lend, hoping for nothing in return. Love your enemies, bless them that curse you, do good to them that hate you, pray for them who would despitefully use you."[1] And my favorite is, "The race is not to the swift, nor the battle to the strong, but of him that shows the greatest mercy!"[2] It is not of him that exercises strong human will, nor of him that runs the fastest race, but the race is won by a heart of mercy.

You see, in order to gain, we must lose our self preservation, self protection and self concerns. To go up, we must be willing to go down. Once again we realize that the first shall be last and he who places himself last, will find himself first.[3]

The second major difference between the two distinctly different consciousnesses is this...

The whole motivation of the human consciousness is based on the fear of loss, lack and limitation. We always see the glass as potentially half empty. We fear what might happen "if." "But what if..." we always say.

We save and plan for the day when we might not have, when we might lose. We suffer under the belief of being limited in our relationships, health, strength, ability, wealth, opportunities, etc. That is why we have perfected the attitude of worry. If we don't have something to worry about, that worries us.

By contrast the whole idea of the Divine Mind of the Eternal Unlimited One is abundance! Abundant life, abundant love, abundant opportunities, abundant acceptance, abundant joy, abundant resources, abundant understanding, wisdom and council...abundance, abundance and more abundance!

"Consider the lilies of the field. They neither toil nor do they spin. Yet Solomon in all his glory was not arrayed like one of these. How much more will your Father clothe you...And seek not what you shall eat or drink, neither be of a doubtful mind...For all these things do the nations of the world seek after...but seek first the kingdom of God (understanding, knowledge, relationship) and all these things will be added to you...abundantly. For where your treasure is there will your heart be also. For I have come to bring to you abundant Life."[4]

The way into the depths of the Mind of God, to see as He sees, to know as He knows, to do as we have been sent to do, comes in no other way except to have the humility to say with Jesus, "I can of my own self do nothing."[5] And to be *willing to give up what we cling to in order to gain what we cannot lose!*

CHAPTER TEN

GOD IS OMNIPRESENT

GOD, BEING PURE SPIRIT, occupies all space and place. There is no place in heaven or earth that the Spirit of God is not occupying.

It is like the air that surrounds us. We live by it, yet we don't see it. We realize the effect it has on us and our complete dependence upon it, yet we cannot touch it. We can feel the wind when it blows, we can see the leaves moving and our hair blowing around...in other words, we can see the effect of what is present, but not see what is causing it.

And so it is with Spirit. I feel it. I realize the impact it has upon me. I realize my total dependence upon it. I know that it fills all space and place and that there is no place or space where it is not present.

We have for centuries been told that hell is a place where God is not. That the experience of hell is experiencing a moment without God. But the Bible contradicts this. It tells us that, "If I make my bed in hell, behold, Thou art there."[1]

Hell is despair and despair is the belief that we will not

see the mercy of God in a particular situation. It is giving up on God, so to speak. Or being convinced that God has abandoned us. But the Eternal Truth here is that God, by His Spirit is everywhere, at all times and present in every human condition.

We can not be bad enough to remove God from our presence. No matter what we are doing or have done, God remains ever present. Goodness surrounds us, whether we realize it or not. Generally it is either ignorance or guilt that keeps us from a constant realization of the presence of God.

God knows no vacuum. If we remove from our mind a thought that has kept us from realizing the Presence of Spirit, then because we have provided space for it, Spirit will move into that space provided. *It will appear in whatever way or form that will correct the human condition.*

Once when I was leaving a particular religious group under quite a bit of strain and duress, one of the leaders of the group declared that if I walked out I would be walking away from God! At the time I was very young and still quite impressionable concerning the things of God, so what she said really rocked me. I thought for a moment and suddenly knew that there was *no place that God was not occupying.*

Therefore there was no place which was not occupied by Love, comfort, protection, direction, peace, etc. In the worst of human conditions, if you are there, then God is there... for He "tabernacles with men"[2] and is the life of all men.

You are sent to this human scene as the Divine Influence upon all human conditions!

If you can remember this when situations arise that are adverse and threatening, you will remain calm and confident and assured knowing that because you stand there, God is there to influence the entire situation for good. You will be able to remain quiet, watchful and listening. Soon the whole circumstance will appear to the glory of God. Goodness, order and peace will prevail. This is true for whatever human condition you might see yourself entangled, whether ill-health, attack from another, sudden loss of anything, etc.

This is true even if, by your judgment, you were the one responsible for the problem in the first place. Remember that God is not reactive. His constant, immutable nature cannot be altered by what man does or fails to do. Whenever the presence of God is realized, even if for only a moment, the nature of God takes over, and all things appear in Divine Order.

CHAPTER ELEVEN

GOD IS DIVINE ORDER

In GENESIS IT IS WRITTEN that under no condition will there ever be a change in the "...winter and springtime, seed time and harvest, day and night, cold and heat."[1]

Because these proceed from an unchangeable nature, they remain perpetual and intact as a manifestation of that nature.

All things that appear in the world of the visible began as a thought. The worlds were framed by the word of God, but that word began as a thought in the Mind of God... otherwise referred to as an image, coming from the word imagination.

Thoughts are the most powerful force in our world. We are unfortunately so very ignorant of this and therefore, we unknowingly think and speak in such a way as to unleash the darkest night upon ourselves! Our very thoughts and words hang us.

This is what is referred to in the Commandments as having a "graven image." A graven image is not simply a piece of gold or silver, a statue or a picture that man may worship, as religion tells us. "Thou shall not make unto thyself any graven image"[2] means that we should be careful what we allow to reside within our thoughts. Whatever is *engraved* in the imagination of our minds will appear in the world of form.

If we don't like what we are experiencing, we need to pray to know what *thought* we are holding that is contrary to the absolute truth...a graven image.

Disease begins as a thought. Not a thought about a particular disease, but an atmosphere of thought that *sees* a world of dis-ease, with confusion ruling and chaos reigning.

In this atmosphere of thought we do not see, nor do we expect to see, goodness (God) ruling His creation in Love and Divine Order. We see circumstances ruling. We see situations ruling. We see ignorance ruling. We see ourselves as being entirely governed by the law of chance.

We see ourselves as mere mortals, vulnerable and fragile within the confines of the bodies that we wear. We have forgotten who formed the body and whose Life gives order, harmony, strength and intelligence to the body. We have forgotten that we have been called the "light of the world!"[3]

We must begin to think of ourselves first as a spiritual being. Children of the Light. The absolute Divine Order here is that *it is the Spirit that determines the physical.* The physical should never be allowed to rule and govern. As soon as we fall into that state of confusion, chaos rules, darkness rules. We become as a runaway train, with no control, no order, no balance, no harmony. And that is disease.

Disease of the mind, disease of the home, the family, the purse, the workplace. Never should the thing created usurp the authority over that which created it.

Therefore the body does not determine the Life. It is the Life which determines the condition of the body.

One only needs to look out upon the world that is formed to realize the undeniable order of all things. The seasons, the stars and planets and galaxies. Look at the animals, the world of insects, the ants and bees.

Look at the intrinsic beauty and harmony of the human body functioning in Divine Order, without one single human being telling it what to do, when, or how! Imagine! In this day of human intervention into every aspect of life, where we are convinced that the normal function of the body simply cannot continue without some pill or some human interfering with its natural order!

Look at the heavens above you. The same stars appear in the same order as they appeared when the worlds were framed. The seasons come and go. The night always gives way to the daylight. All the creatures know whether they are day creatures or night creatures. This never changes. Perfect order from the perfect Mind of perfect Goodness!

Ecclesiastes says this: "One generation passes away and another generation comes...The sun arises and the sun goes down...the wind goes toward the south and turns about to the north, and the wind returns again according to its circuits. All rivers run into the sea, unto the place from where they come, there the rivers return again."[4]

This is a beautiful description of absolute Divine Order.

We need to ask ourselves one question here. Is, somehow and for some reason, the human body exempt from this Principle of the nature of God? Is everything that God has made still under the absolute, sovereign authority of Divine Order except the human body?

Are we the only aspect of creation that needs the help of man to maintain order? Of pills and checkups and x-rays and exams?

Have we somewhere along the way "bought into" something very strange and insane here? Isn't this about the worst case of graven imagery that you have ever heard?

At what point did we give over the Divine Order of our bodies to mere men, to strangers? At what point did we begin to be told and believe that our God-created bodies were victims of 'chance and probability?' Who led us to believe that we were vulnerable to change and confusion and disorder? Because we have certainly bought the picture...hook, line and sinker!

Now we are convinced that we cannot survive without human intervention. And what we believe we experience. Now we only have to believe what we are seeing to reinforce this strange imagery. But when the Christ shall arise in our hearts, "We will not judge after the seeing of our eyes. We will instead judge according to truth and what is eternally right."[5] When our judgments change and our beliefs begin to line up with what is eternally true, then will our experiences change.

No matter what field of science we pursue on this earth, (biology, zoology, botany, astronomy, physics, chemistry, etc.) the one factor that is always present in every facet of life is the Principle of Divine Order.

The question might arise in your mind, what about the diseases we see in nature with the animals, the plants and other manifestations of Life? The answer is found in these words. "All creation groans and travails in pain together waiting for the manifestation of the sons of God." Another translation puts it this way, "All creation stands on its tip-toes waiting for the sons of God to appear."[6]

The Divine Order is that *man* be the "crowning glory of creation." It is man who was given the command to, "Go and take dominion over the earth and subdue it."

We are to subdue it by self-sacrificing love and care for the earth that was given to us for our needs.

But we are also to subdue it by the knowledge of the truth. As we perceive life to be, so is everything under our dominion governed. If we live in disorder and confusion of thought, fearful under the law of chance, so will the rest of creation appear. As we begin to come out of our fog of insanity, lethargy, and selfishness, remembering who we are and why we were sent here...the creatures, the vegetation, the remainder of all creation will respond. No wonder they await our appearing!

SECTION THREE

INTRODUCTION

MANY IDEAS AND UNDERSTANDINGS presented here seem, on surface contact, to be in direct contrast to the teachings of the Bible. This is not true. What is true is that they differ radically from the religious teachings *about* the Bible writings to date.

Paul said that the "letter of the writings will bring death, but interpreting the writings according to the Spirit of Truth will bring Life."[1] Heretofore religion has taught surface interpretations that have been the basic cause of human suffering and death. A deeper look at the same writings will reveal a much different vision and allow for a shift into Life.

Because of the confusion and contradictions of teachings from the Bible, many have thrown the Bible away as a source of truth and comfort. This saddens me deeply. It is my hope and desire that by bringing to light the spiritual significance of the Bible these same people will re-discover a love for it and a confidence in the consistency of the words and understandings. Remember that it was *written by* the

Spirit of Truth, to be interrupted only by the same Spirit. As we lean upon this Spirit for unfolding understandings, we will begin to develop a whole new relationship with the Bible and with the God of the Bible.

CHAPTER ONE

THE TWO COVENANTS

A COVENANT IS A CONTRACT between two parties, or individuals. It is valid only so long as both parties keep their promise, or fulfill their part of the agreement.

For the sake of clarity here I will call the Old Testament a contract that God made with man. It has also been referred to as the Old Covenant. This contract is the basis of the entire Old Testament. The New Testament, or covenant, is the entering in of a new contract between God and man, needed because man was self-destructing under the burden of the first.

Admittedly this may be a lot of information for the average person who is not really familiar with the Bible. But if you understand this, you will see clearly why suffering exists, why we think it is legitimate or necessary and how man began to view God in such a misrepresented manner. Most importantly, you will understand the way that has been provided for us to climb out from under the rubble of this whole deadly scenario.

Remember that understanding is progressive. There was a time that man didn't even know not to kill one another! The human consciousness was so lost in the darkness of its own reasonings and not yet able to perceive a Sovereign God, much less the nature of God to be Love. Survival of the fittest was the order of the day.

Before Abraham, man looked to many gods for whatever was his need at the time. At least he understood that *something* governed creation. With the revelation given to Abraham came the knowledge of one God governing all, and the Life of it all.

However, that seemed to do little to influence the lawlessness of mankind. That is, until Moses received "the law" by which man was to live. It gave mankind boundaries of behavior which he needed to govern himself...*until he progressed enough in his relationship with God where he would no longer need an external list of laws.*[1]

This event took place immediately after the children of Israel left the bondage of Egypt and began their long trek through the wilderness, toward the Promised Land.

Always when Egypt appears in the Bible it refers to the extreme darkness of the human consciousness, a consciousness of terrible slavery and hard bondage to the beliefs of the world. Egypt represents the many ideas and imaginations that we have created and then are subsequently forced to serve under. We then become bound to that which we have believed.

Man was unable to know God...so great was his confusion. So God gave man a standard to live by, which would enable him to find some degree of order. This is not only the Ten Commandments but the entire Levitical law, as well. These standards are enforced by consequences of "rewards and punishments."

It is stated that the *fulfillment of the law is love*.[2] What this means is that when man is filled with the nature of God...which is Love...he does not need the law, for he is *by nature* the fulfillment of it. It is important that we understand this.

The contract that God made with His people was that if they kept this law they would live and receive many blessings. But if they failed to keep the law, they would suffer many tragedies and finally die. Since it was not yet developed within their nature to do it automatically, they labored and strove day and night to fulfill it...and of course, since it was not yet developed within their nature, they failed.

Four thousand years went by with the promise of a new contract. Finally with the advent of Jesus, a new contract or covenant was introduced to mankind and established. This is referred to as the New Testament.

And this is the new covenant that Jesus introduced to man..."*Behold, I will pour my Spirit out upon you. It will over take you and consume you. By my Spirit you will know a new nature...I will write it upon your heart. This new nature will cause you to be able to fulfill the entire law.*" It will be the nature of Love and Mercy. And because of it, you

*will automatically become the fulfillment of the law. You will
not need to strive to become something...for you will realize that you already are that which you have been striving to
become. You cannot fail.³*

This is the true definition and activity of *grace...*

*God, by His Spirit, doing what man, by his efforts, cannot
do.*⁴

This new covenant is to be carried out by *grace alone,*
no longer by the sweat and toil of man's efforts to please
God by keeping a standard of laws. When this "new" covenant appeared, the old was done away.⁵ Why? Because now
the Spirit of God, Itself, would be living the life of man and
fulfilling the demands of its own nature within man!

Human effort and 'striving to gain' is an
acknowledgement that we do not understand who we are
and what is the eternal truth of our existence. Human
effort to achieve anything spiritually is a declaration that
we do not understand grace. It is the opposite of grace. When
we fall back into human effort to achieve anything with
God, we are putting ourselves back under the old covenant,
with its laws and punishments.

"By grace" you already are who you are.

"By grace" you will come to know and understand the
true nature of God and be found as Him.⁶

"By grace" you will overcome whatever obstacle seems
to be in your path; that is anything that denies who you are
and what God is in your life.

"By grace" means then the Spirit and activity and Presence and power of God *alone will do whatever is necessary at any given time and circumstance.*

Sounds wonderful, doesn't it? But now here is the problem.

We are still living under the law. We are not accepting the reality that Jesus came to show us and to teach us. We are still trying to be worthy…trying to earn something from God. We are still trying to "please God" so as not to incur the wrath that we believe will follow our failures.

We are still striving under the burden of a *personal sense of responsibility* for our lives. We do not know that there is but One Life… and God is, by His Spirit, living that Life *within and through* each facet of creation, including us. Especially us! "For of Him and through Him and to Him are all things."[7]

We are not living in and out from this "new nature."

We don't see ourselves as Love and Mercy and we don't see anyone else as that either.

And yet we are told that this Spirit is the "true Light which lights every man born into this world."[8] But we are still trying to earn it *as though it doesn't already exist.*

We are told that we are the light of the world, but we don't believe it.

We are told that "of His fullness have we all received"[9] …not *will* receive, but *have* received. But we don't believe it.

We are told that we *have been* translated out from the

kingdom of darkness (human consciousness) into the kingdom of His dear Son[10] (Divine Life being manifested in the earth), but we don't believe it either.

We are told that "He is the Father of lights (which we are) with whom there is no shadow of turning...no changing."[11]

We still act as though we need to earn something...but sadly never believing that we really will. This is what religion is saying and we have all, like sheep led to the slaughter, bought into it.

But this directly contradicts what the Spirit of God says and what Jesus came to teach us. So why have we not accepted it, and why are they still teaching the old but declaring that the new has come? The answer is simple. We believe what we are seeing...and see what we are believing. We are doing exactly what Jesus said not to do and that is to judge according to outward appearances. Once again, we are told to "judge righteously."[12]

And once again, righteous judgment is simply that we choose to judge and believe that we are what He has made us to be. That we are a fulfillment of the law. That we are the personification of Love and Mercy. And that *so is everyone else*!

We must first believe it because it is true...then and only then, we will see it. That is faith. Believing what is true, in spite of what our eyes see or our hearts interpret.

CHAPTER TWO

HOW TO LIVE IN
THE NEW COVENANT

REMEMBER THE NEW COVENANT SAYS that the Spirit of God will live this life for you, so that you will always, by the nature of that Spirit, live righteously. All good will be your lot in life. Only blessings and the abundance of everything that God is, will be your portion forever.

However if we choose to remain within the confines of the old law, we will continue to suffer from our own sense of futility and failure.

So, how do we enter into this contract? *We learn to listen.* We learn to block out the constant chatter and advice of Babylonish nonsense. We stop letting every desire and whim rule our decisions. We stop being carried along day after day by the "wisdom" of men. We stop looking to the "learned" for direction and advice.

Read the words of the prophet Isaiah with me:

"Woe unto the rebellious children, says the Lord, who take counsel, but not by me...that walk to go down to Egypt (human ways and means) for help, but have not asked at my mouth.

They strengthen themselves in the strength of Pharaoh, and trust in the shadow of Egypt. (This is referring to trusting in the ways and means that the whole world follows after.) Therefore will the strength of Pharaoh be your shame and the trust in the shadow of Egypt be your confusion. They were all ashamed of a people that could not profit them, nor be a help to them, but a shame.

For those who you turn to for help, shall help in vain, and to no purpose."

"Woe unto them who put their trust in the horses, because they are many, and chariots, because they are strong. (This is judging that the way of the world, that which men follow after, is stronger and more powerful than the way of God.) For the Egyptians are men and not God and their horses flesh and not spirit."[1]

Now make no mistake, it is not God who has caused the failure and the subsequent suffering that is incurred when we "go our own way." But we have put ourselves back under "success by human effort" living, (or the law of sowing and reaping, cause and effect,) which brings about our own suffering.

So now hear what follows:

"Therefore have I cried out to them concerning this. Their strength is to *sit still*. In returning and rest shall you be saved from this evil...in quietness and confidence shall be your strength."[2]

We must learn to listen. To let the Spirit of wisdom and counsel and direction lead out in every situation, in every decision that needs to be made. We must remember that our life is not our own. There is one Life and we are manifestations of that Life.

We were created with a purpose. We were *sent* with a purpose that needs to be fulfilled. Since we have no idea what that is, we cannot by our own wisdom make it happen.

We don't know what is ahead in our future, therefore, how can we make wise choices without knowing the whole picture? We don't know what will happen one hour from now, much less the rest of our lives! It is probably good that we don't have a pre-programmed road map of our lives...we would never learn to listen and trust the answers that come.

Learning to listen is also referred to as "waiting" for the word of God. Waiting is definitely not passive here. It is most active. It requires more focus and commitment than anything else you will probably do the rest of your life. It is hard to sit still, pray and wait when everything in you is screaming, "You better do something fast!" But even so, nothing you do will be as effective, or more beneficial, than 'not doing'...but instead waiting for the direction and counsel of Divine mind.

Do not mistake this for denial or ignoring the problem. You are not ignoring it...you are healing it. You are just not doing it the way the whole world declares that you should. So they, in the pride of believing that their way is the only way, tell you that you are "in denial." You would not believe how many times I have heard that in my life! Nor would you believe how many healings I have seen because I didn't listen to such foolish chatter.

So how do we hear the voice of God? Or better put, how do we *feel* the impulse of the Spirit within?

The first step is the hardest. We must let go of any desired outcome. What that means is that we cannot go to God for direction and counsel already predetermining a specific answer. We will never be able to *feel* what the direction is because we will be so clouded in our thoughts, clinging to what we want. *We must trust that God is good and only goodness can come;* we must know the nature of God enough to know that! We cannot direct what should happen or how it should appear. It is enough for us to know that *only the perfection and goodness of God can appear.* For God is good and the whole purpose of God in the Earth is to appear...to be revealed in every single situation and event...that God might be "all in all." That goodness might fill the whole land![3]

We must know that Spirit is always leading and guiding, always speaking and directing. We do not always listen, so we do not always hear. The Spirit of wisdom and counsel and understanding was given to us "to lead and guide us into *all* truth...which truth will always make you free from whatever is challenging you."[4] It is freely available for every occasion.

Listen to Isaiah again when he writes, "And you shall hear a word behind you saying, 'This is the way, walk ye in it,' when you turn to the right hand or to the left."[5]

And when the word comes to you, "the light of the moon shall be as the light of the sun and the light of the sun shall be sevenfold."[6] So great will be the blessing of God upon you.

When you let Spirit lead and rule your life and you learn the wisdom of listening, you can not imagine what your life will be like. "For eye hath not seen, nor has ear heard, all that God has prepared for those who love Him."[7] (To those who trust their lives to His Infinite Wisdom.) "Not my will but Thine be done," becomes easy, actually comfortable, when you realize from your heart that *His will is your will.*[8]

My first daughter, Linda, was always such a deep, spiritually focused child. But she often struggled with turning over her will for a higher, more perfect wisdom. I tried in so many ways to help her see that the mind of God could never do anything but bless her. One day it came to me to say to her, "You share the same heart as God...and God is only Love. *God leads us by the desires of our heart.* It is the Wisdom of God that appears to us *as* our desires. They are the same. You can let go of your tight grip knowing that what you surrender will come back to you in abundance." And that finally settled the matter.

To continue to fear what the "will of God" might be is to be leaning back into the doctrine of a man-like god who rewards and punishes, who might pull the rug out from under us at any given moment! Admittedly, a frightening thought!

The answer from God will never hurt you, or cause you pain. You may walk through some pretty strange places, but He will go before you to make the crooked ways straight. The goodness and abundance of God awaits you for your faithfulness to listen and follow. Every situation will teach you and cause you to rise higher and higher into the Mind and understanding of God. And the end of that road is peace.

CHAPTER THREE

THE SPIRITUAL SIGNIFICANCE OF THE SABBATH

THE WORD SABBATH MEANS "REST." The Sabbath is not a day of the week as most doctrines hold. It is not doing something on a special day. These are traditions of men and while they hold certain significance for some, the true meaning and purpose of the Sabbath is lost. The "rest" of God is found in the quietness of the soul, deep in the enveloping Love of Divine Love Itself.

It is said that God rested after the seventh day of creation. He ceased from His work because it was finished and He was satisfied that it was complete. For us to honor this Sabbath day is for us to also enter into the "rest" of God and stop our struggling as though the work is not finished and something more must be done for us.

We are in the Spirit of the One Life and "all is well." When we know this deep in our hearts, we are content, we are peaceful and we are able then to realize the quiet confidence of Eternal Love as it envelops our hearts.

But when we are facing a specific challenge, a temptation to believe in the power of evil over our lives...and we have forgotten who we are and that "all that needs to be done is already done,"[1] we begin to struggle and fret and worry and run here and there to find the help that we believe we need. We have ceased to "believe" and ceased to "rest."

When these times occur, we would do well to stop! Stop the terrible impulse to "do something." Stop the panic. Stop and remember the One Life and the Spirit of that Life that will "lead and guide you into all truth." [2] It will only be in that place of "rest" that we will be able to know the direction we are to take.

My favorite prayer at such times as these is, "What is it that I have forgotten?" "What is it that I need to know here?" If we are faithful to remain in that place of rest until the answer begins to dawn within our soul, we will *always* find that the One Life is still governing and "all is well." We will find the evil that appeared is no power at all... and that the One Power is still governing in the present perfection of the One Life, regardless of the immediate threat.

A sense of rest and peace is God's gift to us for our security in times of challenge. The traditions of men have us doing something on a special day to honor God. But everyday is the Sabbath when we live in the peace and trust and quietness of Spirit that comes with knowing the truth. This is why Jesus said that "the Sabbath was made for man, and not man for the Sabbath."[3]

When we have developed our sense of the Christ consciousness, whereby everyday we are being led by the wisdom and council of the Spirit, *which is our life*...then we are "keeping holy the Sabbath." Temptations assail us daily to absorb the cares and concerns of situations and human dramas. We must always "remember the Sabbath, to keep it holy." This exercise, this place of peace and assurance, is "given to us" for our joy and the assurance of a peaceful and healthy and fulfilled life. This is the way to live and this is the way to deal with the darkness that so often appears to us in so many varied forms and appearances.

Not long ago I was accompanying my youngest daughter to one of her pre-natal visits. I was anxious to meet her OB doctor, having heard so many nice things about him from her. During the visit his assistant discovered that I had never submitted to a test for cervical cancer. Actually, I had never been to a doctor for any tests or check-ups since my babies were born and had no thought to do so. But for a reason unknown to me at the time I decided to let the test be done that day. I left and returned home, thinking nothing of it again. A few days later I received a call from the doctor's office saying that the test was positive for cervical cancer. They told me that the abnormal cells were quite extensive throughout the cervix and I should come in immediately to talk with the doctor.

Once I realized what was being said to me, I quickly shifted into the spiritual mode of thought. Since I was convinced that I was a child of Light, sent to "undo the works of darkness," and "Nothing shall by any means hurt me,"[4] I concluded that this was simply an evidence of darkness that needed to be dissolved by the shining of the light of truth. I told the nurse that I would not do anything until after my granddaughter was born. This was a very special and sacred time for our family and I wasn't going to allow evil in any shape or form to spoil it. This also was my way of putting her off until I had the chance to pray about the whole thing.

Two of my assistants at the clinic, and very dear friends, were standing beside me when the call came in. I asked them to support me in prayer and not say a word to anyone, not even to speak of this between themselves. They agreed. We are quite cognizant of the power of our words for good or ill, so this was not foreign to them. I determined not to tell anyone in my family either until I had a chance to pray about it, which was pretty much how I always handle problems anyway. The more people who know about specific challenges, the more their fears and concerns cloud up the 'atmosphere of thought,' making extrication from any situation more difficult.

One month later my daughter gave birth to her baby and we were able to rejoice, enjoying every moment of the experience without any gloom hanging over us. Soon we all settled back into our life routines and I began to ask God to prepare space for me to deal with this now.

During my daughter's first post natal visit to her doctor's office, the nurse told her what was going on with me, with the hope that she would have some influence to convince me to return to them for treatment. So now the whole family knew. I agreed to a biopsy where the performing physician described in detail the "masses" that he observed and the 'salt and pepper' scatterings of abnormal cells throughout.

We returned home where we began to quietly but fervently pray. I began to feel the strength of their support and knew it was time to 'press in.' The whole effort took about three days. The house was quiet, the atmosphere was focused, but confident. I stayed awake all night the first night, reading and remembering who I am, why I have come here and simply feeling the Presence of Divine Love. This enabled me to gain entrance into the "Sabbath rest," which I knew would allow space for God to speak. This entering into the "rest" allowed all anxiety to subside, and the realization of Love began to fill my heart.

This challenge came after years of studying, questioning, learning and seeing thousands of irrefutable proofs of the truths I was being taught. I determined to allow this temple of my soul to be filled with the Presence and power of the glory of God. It replaced the lingering unrest, fear and dread, and total distortion of truth, that the dark suggestions of the human consciousness always carries.

My foundation of thought began with remembering what I already knew to be true, setting the cornerstone for the Holy Spirit to begin to build whatever new understandings it would.

I remembered that I am a child of Light, not a result of a random DNA, nor the will of my parents.

I remembered that I was not dealing with disease. But instead, I was dealing with Divine Love, for Love is omnipresent...the knowledge of which cancels any place or space for evil to exist.

I remembered that I was sent to this earthly existence, not to seek my own self interests, not to preserve this mortal experience, but to fulfill the purpose of God. And to let the expression of truth, harmony and perfection have the freedom to appear in any given situation.

I remembered that my life is 'not my own.'[5] I do not have an individual life, separate and apart from the One Life that is God...or the one expression of that Life, which is called the Christ. ("When Christ, *who is your life* shall appear...")[6]

I remembered that the reason we, as the light, have appeared in this earthy form was to 'undo the works of darkness'... and how could we do this unless we come face to face with it?

I remembered that the will and purpose of God is to reveal His glory. That is, to appear as the Light, harmony, beauty and perfection to every appearance of darkness.

I remembered that this was really not about me at all!

Knowing all this with all my heart, I was able to surrender to the grace that I knew must flow through my soul and my mind, for only by grace, the activity of Spirit, would this darkness be resolved and the light of the Glory of God be revealed.

The next morning I received a call from Kay, one of the two friends who stood beside me when I first received the call. She also had been praying and during this time heard a word over and over again in her mind, giving her impulse to look up the definition in the dictionary. The word was "disdain." The first definition was the common one, "to look at someone with condescending contempt, from an ignoble mind." But the second listed definition was what prompted her to call me. It said, "A passionate, forceful hatred of evil from a noble mind." We both realized that this was declaring that the Christ, (the Spirit of God revealed through creation) *stood before this evil*, not only in our behalf, but in behalf of the appearing of the harmony and perfection of God, replacing the human beliefs with the Divine Mind.

Evil loves to declare its right to exist, to be feared and honored as a power to contend with. It loves to usurp its authority over the authority of Eternal Life and immense Love. It declares darkness to be stronger than light, hate to be stronger than love, confusion to be stronger than order, lies to be stronger than truth. But here was the Christ, declaring its power, its presence, its authority, its truth.

When I heard those words, I felt a definite shift in consciousness and realized that I had just entered into the "rest" of the Sabbath. Peace and assurance flooded my soul. I felt an overwhelming sense of gratitude and knew I would be "led" as to what I should do, if anything. I knew that no matter what I must face, I was going to be okay. Everything was going to be okay!

The next day while at the clinic, I was climbing into the chamber of the hyperbaric oxygen unit to arrange something for a patient when I suddenly had a very definite and intense *vision* of a wolf standing before me, fierce and aggressive, with its eyes yellow and slanted, baring its teeth. This animal was in "attack mode!" Instantly the form of a shepherd jumped between us. Facing the wolf, I could see the back of his robe-like garment with a rope tied about his waist. His legs were spread, his arms raised and a cat-ofnine-tails whip was in his right hand. He was defending his lamb. It all happened so fast when I heard the words, "The wolf is at the door. But don't worry, Michele, *I am the door!*"

With those words the vision vanished. Melissa, my other friend who was with me at the first phone call, was also in the chamber behind me. I turned to her and collapsed, stunned and in tears. I kept repeating, "Melissa, the wolf is at the door, but He is the door!" Over and over again I said those words, crying so hard she could barely understand me. I had never felt such love in all my life. Patiently she sat with me, not knowing what could have prompted this sudden emotion, and held my hand until the impact of the whole experience began to subside. I was telling her the vision when the phone rang. It was the doctor's office with the report from the biopsy. I cannot tell you how peaceful I was taking that phone call. It may as well have been a weather report! They told me what I expected to hear. There was no sign, no observable indication of anything wrong at all. Later I asked the doctor what he thought of it all. He had just finished reading my first book, *Of Monkeys and Dragons, Freedom from the Tyranny of Disease,* so he smiled and said, "I would have expected nothing less!"

This is the result of knowing the truth, of entering into the rest of God, which comes from believing what you have come to know. This is the clear result of the free flow of *grace,* fulfilling the will of God, and bringing harmony to every human event. It is available for everyone right now, it is the reason that we exist here in this human form.

Chapter Four

THE LAW OF SOWING AND REAPING

Now the natural law, the law of cause and effect which governs the earth, is also called the law of sowing and reaping as we have mentioned earlier. "Whatsoever you sow, that shall you also reap." This *is* the law of Moses. If you do good, you can expect goodness. If on the other hand, you do evil, you can expect that will also return to you. This doesn't only apply to what we *do*. What we are *not* told is that if we even *believe* in the power of evil to rule indiscriminately, it will. If, on the other hand, we believe that there is only One Power, and that is the power and omnipresence of Goodness ruling its creation, we will also reap that expectation. According to the deepest expectations of our consciousness, so we experience.

The inability of man to fulfill that original law caused mankind to live under the realization of defeat, failure and *expectation of punishment*...some sort of suffering.

It makes us critical of ourselves and everyone else. It is the basis and platform of all judgment.

This law is the cause of all disease, poverty, sadness, tears, and pain in the earth. It is the cause of death. This is the infamous *karma* that we hear so much about. A bottomless pit. The reason for suffering and human anguish. What we *don't hear* is that we were intended to *transcend* the law of karma. Under this law we are motivated by fear. Fear of punishment. This is the lowest form of motivation. Whereas love for God, and living out from that love as our own nature, is the highest form of motivation.

We have believed that it is God who punishes us, when in fact *it is our own transgression of our conscience and the expectation of punishment that draws our suffering.* Living under the law itself, and judging ourselves and everyone else according to that law, is enough to secure the untoward effects of the law to us.

The natural law governs the natural man. But because man could not keep that law...*a new way was implemented.* This is called the new covenant, of which we have spoken... that God would do, by his Spirit which resides within man, that which man could not do separate from the activity of that Spirit. "Now unto him who is able to do *exceedingly abundantly* above all that we ask *or think,* according to the power *that works within us.*"[1]

God would reveal to man his true relationship with his Creator. He would cause man to see who he really is in the eternal *oneness* of his relationship with God. Biblically this is called the *new creation,*[2]...one that God could live through and demonstrate His marvelous nature. While this is referred to as a "new" creation, it is actually the creation as it was known by Divine Mind since "before the foundation of the world."[3] That God, by his Spirit, would live and govern and *be* the life of everything formed. Once again the definition of living by grace.

You can image that whatever God lived through, animated, and directed...would be beyond description. It would never know misery, fear or darkness of any sort. It would walk in the light of the glory of God. Happiness, joy and abundance would be its *only expectation. No one would or could ever be sick.* Tears would only be those of joy and gladness and gratitude. "For of him and to him and through him are all things."[4]

Now how do we regain that which we have forgotten? How do we move away from the *futile efforts of man* to become something that we *already* are?

The only prerequisite would be that we *realize* that we cannot keep this law (and therefore cannot avoid the suffering that follows.) And that we *stop trying.* Let go of *human effort* to know, to do and to be.

Our job is to *lean into the Spirit,* to allow it to live its life through us. Allow it to keep the law of Love which is the fulfillment of the natural law. We can never really be separated from this Love, which "freely gives us all things."[5] We must live in the *awareness* of the Spirit of Divine Life and Eternal Love always filling our being and motivating our existence. We must let it have the uninterrupted expression that it desires.

This is referred to as *The Law of the Spirit of Life.*

CHAPTER FIVE

THE LAW OF THE SPIRIT OF LIFE

*"For the law of the Spirit of Life has made
me free from the law of sin and death."*[1]

C AN WE TRANSCEND THE NATURAL LAW of sowing and reaping, cause and effect? Yes, we can. But there is only one way to do this and that is to find, and place ourselves under a *higher law*. The Bible refers to this new law as the "law of the Spirit of Life."

Entering into this new law, or understanding, will free us from the effects of the law of cause and effect, from the whole karmic influence. Think of it! A way has been provided for mankind to live above all the suffering and tragedies, pains and fears, which have enslaved us since time began. One can only wonder, since this has been recorded for two thousand years, why are we not hearing about it from the day we are born? Why are we still living under a way of thought which continues to cause us the very sufferings that we strive so hard to be free from? For the law of cause and effect (with all of its punishments and sufferings) will continue to govern the "natural" man until he chooses to transcend this law. And how can we choose unless we are made aware of another option?

We can only transcend this whole arena by the entering in of a new understanding, a new revelation, an entirely new and different way of seeing life. And this has been freely provided for us, both the knowledge of it and the power to live it.

୶

To understand the mind of God, in contrast to the "doctrines of men," we must first divest ourselves of any beliefs or understandings previously held. We can do this simply by being willing to learn something new... to have no particular investment in anything previously held as true or sacred to us. When we want to know the truth more than we want to breathe...that's a good start!

In the Old Testament there are many, sometimes strange laws that God gave to Moses to govern the children of Israel. One was, as the people traveled through the "wilderness experience," heading towards the "promised land," they were not to build any houses, temples or any other permanent structures along the way. They were to live in tents only. This was so that whenever the Spirit of God moved upon them to begin to travel again, they would not be reluctant to do so because they had become so comfortable where they were.

Just so are we encouraged, while we travel on to the "promised land" of the "true knowledge of the Eternal One" and the goodness that that promises us, not to "build a shrine" to any particular doctrine, person, place, or comfort zone. We should always be ready to "hear" and respond, and to "move on" in our understanding, when directed.

This, then, is the promise given to us, and the clear understanding of the simplicity of entering into it. This is the understanding of the Law of the Spirit of Life.

There is a Spirit of Life. It is what gives life to all living things. There is One Spirit and therefore One Life. It is the same life for a plant as it is for an insect. It is the same Life for a person as it is for a bird. This One Life, not only flows throughout all of its creations, but is what actually formed all the visible formations that we see. Same Life, but different manifestations. *Each manifestation declaring something of the nature of that Spirit of Life.*

Once again, there is a Divine law here that states, "Each seed reproduces after its own kind."[2] So it is with God. "It is He that hath made us and not we ourselves."[3]

As the name God means *good,* so out from the Divine and eternal realm of all *goodness* comes forth all the worlds and universe; all the inhabitants of the earth and the stars, planets and suns in the heavens.

Every living creature, everything that grows...all that we call alive, everything that we see comes from the same source...the one Spirit of Life. It is this Spirit which flows through all life, formed all life, and animates all life.

The book of Job in the Old Testament says this, "The Spirit of God made me and the breath of the Almighty hath given me life."[4] We actually existed before our bodies were formed, in and as this Spirit of Life. Again the book of Job tells us, "...When the foundations of the earth were laid and the morning stars sang together, and all the sons of God shouted for joy."[5]

໒ຉ

Why does this One Life form so many varied formations? Because there are so many facets, so many characteristics of this One Life. Through these varied formations, it describes itself. It expresses itself.

If we had eyes to see and a heart to understand, we would learn to see God everywhere we looked. We would see *goodness and purity and wholeness, immutable order, perpetual perfection everywhere we looked. For all things declare God.* In the New Testament, Paul writes, "For the invisible things of Him, from the creation of the world, are clearly seen, being understood by the things that are made..."[6] And David, the King and poet penned these words, "The heavens declare the glory of God; and the firmament shows His handiwork. Day unto day utters speech, and night unto night shows knowledge. There is no speech nor language, where their voice is not heard. Their words have gone out to the end of the world."[7]

These men realized that they were not *just looking at things* created by God, but at *God Himself*...declaring and describing Himself for all the world to know Him and to enjoy Him.

When the aged Patriarch, Job was searching for the knowledge and wisdom of God, he declared, "Ask now the beasts of the field, and they shall teach thee; and the fowls of the air and they shall tell thee. Or speak to the earth and it shall teach thee; and the fishes of the sea shall declare unto thee."[8] It was no mystery to these men that creation was birthed to manifest and declare and describe its Creator.

From the Mind and heart of the Eternal One there is one grand and glorious, uninterrupted, unchangeable, perpetual, constant perfection...for He is perfect that formed it. It is the One Spirit of Life that breathes and flows throughout it all.

This is the fullness of God. This is the image and likeness from which we have all come.

There is One God, One source of all life and there is One manifestation of the fullness of that Life *and that is called the Son*...the visible expression of the invisible God...also referred to as the Christ.[9] We are not talking about a singular person here, but the total of all, *as the one. Jesus himself declared this in his prayer written throughout chapter 17 of the book of John.*

God sees only Himself in creation...a complete and perfect expression of Himself.

This picture of creation, as God created it and as God sees it, is in direct contrast with the story we have all been told and lived under for 6,000 painful years. It is time that we let go of that story. We must no longer see ourselves as unworthy. We must not see ourselves as worthy either! The whole question of worthiness is not an issue at all. We just are what we are! The object of Divine Love and the expression of Divine Love.

We are the expression of the One Eternal Life. We are *one with all that is.* We must let go of a God whose favor we need to earn. We must let go of a remote place, called heaven, which we also need to earn. For the kingdom of heaven is and always has been within us.

We must just feel Love and loved.

The law, with all its rules and punishments for transgressing those rules, is dead![10]

When we enter into the space of Divine Love, when we allow Love to live its Life *as us,* when we allow Love to be our nature...all the rules are automatically fulfilled by just *loving and being Love.* We are loving and being Love by not needing to defend ourselves; by not needing to retaliate; by not wanting to 'get more' than the next guy...but by just loving and *being Love;* by not judging others according to outward appearances; by not judging our own actions and thoughts by outward appearances...but by knowing that any darkness that we see is not us at all. Nor is it the other guy at all. It is just darkness...only darkness. And that darkness will flee as soon as we are moving in and as Love! Just as soon as we choose to see Love as the other guy, or as ourselves...instead of seeing a sinning mortal!

We must quit giving evil power to act, to be. It is just darkness. A space Love needs to fill...and we are that Love. So when we stand, *being Love* in the face of any darkness... the darkness goes. It cannot remain in the presence of Divine Love. Even the physical appearance of disease will not be able to remain in that sacred Presence.

We have come here to cause the darkness to go...not to judge it.

Not to condone it...not to allow it...but not to condemn it

either. Just to make it go; by recognizing that there is only Divine Life and Divine Love everywhere and as everyone.

So all that being said, from where does disease and other evils arise? From a misunderstanding of truth. When truth is not seen or understood, man made doctrines are created!

Disease, and all other manifestations of evil, *is simply a place and space* (in consciousness only) *where we* (coming from a darkened human perception of life) *have not yet perceived that we are a part of the One Life.* Isn't all human suffering a place where we have "believed and judged evil to exist?" Isn't it true that when we stand in the dark, the images we see are interpreted from our imagination or experiences?

I remember a story of a man who was watching the apartment of his friend who was going to be away for awhile. He lived just across the alley, so it was easy for him to keep an eye out for the safety of his friend's apartment. One night he saw a man standing in the alley right near the back door of the apartment! The man had on a hat and overcoat, and just stood for the longest time with his hands in his pockets. This frightened the man so much that he finally called the police. When the police arrived with lights blazing, it was easy to see immediately that what the man was seeing was not evil, but only the trash cans in the dim shadows of the moonlight.

From birth to death we are trained to fear, look for and expect evil in the form of disease. We are taught to expect failure of the body to maintain health and vigor as we grow older. We are trained to see evil in another person, perhaps who might try to steal from us, or take advantage of us for their own gain. We are plagued by songs on the airways of those who we depended upon, who now have disappointed us, deceived us, left us, destroyed us, etc. We are afraid of accidents, weather, seasonal changes, plants, trees, flowers, animals, and insects. We never have enough, and are always in fear of losing what meager portions we do have. We are looking at the human experience from the eyes of death. This is the veil we spoke of earlier.

Disease is not the enemy...but the taught and trained human consciousness which perceives evil. The human consciousness, the present human awareness, is the only thing we need to be delivered from. When that is cleared, the light of the glory of the One Life appears and all things appear different. This is why Jesus said time and again..."Don't judge!" Your judgment is only coming from what you have learned. You are seeing what is being believed! You have heard the saying, "Seeing is believing?" What it ought to say is "believing is seeing!"

Probably the best definition of the human consciousness is this:

"An imagery of popular belief; floating with the popular current of mortal thought without questioning the reliability of its conclusions...so that we do what others do, believe what others believe and say what others say... therefore experience what others experience!"

The Bible has a neat word for this concept. We spoke of it earlier. It is called Babylon, and it comes from the root word, "to babble." It first appears in the Old Testament with the story of the Tower of Babel.[11] The "learned and brilliant men" of those days decided to build a tower to reach heaven. This is no different than all the religious doctrines and traditions of men, created by men, to "reach heaven" or attain to the blessings they seek. Because this was not an effort which had its origin from God, it failed. Just as modern religion and science has failed to supply us with either freedom from suffering or any true knowledge or understanding of the source of it all.

It is said that God looked at what man had created (tower of Babel) from his *imagination* and decided to "confound the language and words of men so that all their words and understandings would be forever confounded." Confused, convoluted and contradictory! Hence, babbling! Pretty much what we have been listening to throughout the ages.

Unless something comes from the Spirit of Life, it simply has no life within it. It cannot bring forth life or understanding or truth! All the efforts of men to reach and please God…to try to earn favor or blessings…are all experiencing Babylon. Why? Because if we are who He says we are…we are already one with God and need not try to earn anything at all. To *try* then, is to deny this truth and see ourselves separate and apart from our true life.

Later the children of Israel were taken into captivity by the Babylonians! Unfortunately, as a *collective* human consciousness, we remain in captivity to this human consciousness to this day. But the promise is that the veil is lifted and Babylon is fallen. What remains when this is completed in our experience is the *full expression of the Mind of God.*

Living Life no longer in fear and unworthiness, but in joy and freedom and perpetual gladness.

Adam and Eve had two sons, Cain and Abel.[12] Again, whether you believe this literally or see it as an allegory makes no difference here. These two sons are, symbolically speaking, a declaration of the two natures of mankind: one, the natural man, without light and understanding birthed yet within his soul; the other, the Christ of God, the expression of all that God is.

Cain, feeling a separation from the Spirit, or Life of God, worked to please God, in order to be found acceptable. It says he toiled by the sweat of his brow tilling the earth (his soul) to bring forth fruit that would be worthy to God, that He might accept him. But God rejected Cain's sacrifice and efforts. Why? Because they came from a mind that did not see its present perfection and oneness with the Spirit of God. So it tried to bridge that gap by human efforts to please God. Not realizing its own present worthiness, it tried to become worthy. This, as we have sadly seen for 6,000 years of man, will never bring us into the consciousness of the Christ.

Abel, on the other hand, symbolic of the soul of man knitted to the Life of God as One, offered God a Lamb...and that offering was acceptable to God. The lamb always refers to the Christ nature. It is obedient, submitted and totally trusting. It has no defense, for it sees no need for defense. The consciousness of its own life is lost in the oneness it feels with its Shepherd. Abel knew who he was and from where he came.

In jealousy, Cain killed his brother, Abel. This is symbolic of the generations of darkness that would cover the earth, a period when it would appear that evil had overcome any sense of the presence of good...when man would have no understanding of who he is and the Life that he lives. The third son born to Adam and Eve, Seth, symbolizes the coming of a "new creation," revealed two thousand years ago... man in full awareness of his heritage and his strength. Man realizing he need do nothing to earn or reach for this, for this is who he truly is...a new creation.

The undeniable truth is that nothing can truly alter what is eternal. We can believe we are fragile and consigned to disease and intolerable suffering, we can listen to those who teach this and then change the truth of God to fit their doctrines. We can worship at the altar of modern science and medicine that declares we come from matter only and are subject to all the ills thereof. We can believe that we live under the law of chance, a roll of the dice. All this then will we experience. But not because it is the immutable truth of God and us in His image, manifesting His glory, but because we see it, and think it is so.

To live in the conscious awareness of being in the One Life, inseparable and undefiled...*is* the Law of the Spirit of Life that makes us free from the law of sin, sickness and death.

Chapter Six

NEW CREATURE IN CHRIST

O<small>NCE WHEN</small> I <small>WAS ABOUT</small> 26 <small>YEARS OLD</small> and had been a heavy smoker for at least 8 years, I felt strongly that it was time for me to stop the habit. I labored under the belief that the habit 'had me.' I believed, heart and soul, that I was enslaved by those cigarettes and that it would take 'a miracle' to get me to quit. Needless to say, I had set myself up for sure failure with such a mind-set. The more power and energy I gave to that thought, the bigger the battle for me. Pretty soon I had in my mind a mountain to overcome about the size of Mt. Everest.

Every day I would try to stop smoking. I threw away more packs of cigarettes than I could count, but always right after I finished smoking one. By the time I felt the need for another cigarette they were gone. Then in utter failure I would drive to the store to buy another pack. Sometimes after throwing them out of the car window, hours later I would find myself rummaging in the tall weeds on the side of the road for my lost pack of cigarettes. Defeated and condemned, I cried and prayed for God to 'take away' my desire for the cigarettes. Finally, it happened! Every time I started to smoke I felt as though I would throw up. The discomfort of the nausea far outweighed the enjoyment of a cigarette, so very soon I stopped smoking.

But a few weeks later when some human drama had wrapped itself around my life, I started again. I guess I thought that smoking would somehow help me get through it. Now I was really condemned! Here God had delivered me and now I was back at it again! Surely, in disgust, He would leave me to figure it out on my own this time! (Such was my pathetic belief of the harshness of the nature of God.)

Finally one day while sitting in my overstuffed chair reading my Bible, with one leg draped over the arm of the chair and a cigarette in my hand, I came across a scripture in II Corinthians 5:17 and it read, "For you are a new creature in Christ, old things are passed away and all things are become new...and all things are of God." It struck me like lightening. If I really was a new creature in Christ and all that is of the old is gone, then would this new creature be smoking? Had this new creature ever smoked? If this new creature would not begin such a habit and had never done so, then why, I reasoned, would I want to start it now? Down and out went the cigarette and I never picked one up again. Several times for the next few days I would repeat those questions to myself and the desire would leave. Would this Life of Christ have a desire for this?

Years later, I had an occasion to remember this truth

again. As a graduate, pediatric ICU nurse, I was stuck in an elevator for several hours with a newborn who had just died of a congenital heart condition. From that experience on I never got into an elevator alone. I developed a paralyzing fear of being trapped inside and alone. It was nothing for me to walk up 15 to 20 flights of stairs if necessary to avoid an elevator. Thirty years later I wanted to experience a hyperbaric oxygen treatment and knew that to do so meant that I had to climb into a chamber alone and remain there with the door sealed for almost two hours. Given my history, I knew I was fooling myself to think I could manage it.

Suddenly I found myself furious at such a dominating fear. I rose up inside and with all the strength of the Christ Life and the power of the word, I declared out loud, "I do not give my consent to this unreasonable fear!" Immediately a very cynical and sneering thought appeared saying, "Why not? You have always given me your consent?" At first I thought it had me again, but then I knew that the real I, the eternal, divine Life of God had never given consent to such nonsense and as soon as I said it, with all the conviction of eternity behind those words, it left.

Twenty minutes later and without a care or concern, I entered the chamber, let them seal the door and remained in perfect peace throughout the entire treatment. I have easily entered elevators alone since that experience as well.

You see, as long as I gave a reason for the fear to be there, it remained. As long as I gave it a history, such as my unfortunate experience with the baby, it remained. Once I quit identifying as the mortal with the drama and began to realize my identity as the eternal Life of Christ...knowing that this Life would never entertain such hysterical fears...the healing or correction occurred.

We can apply this to the health and wholeness of our lives and bodies as we remember that we are "in Christ." As such we can no more experience such educated, hysterical madness as disease than could an elephant fly! We have ignorantly given our consent to such tragedy, but this can end at this very moment. As we withdraw our consent to such beliefs, declaring and knowing the truth of our being, "hid in Christ in God,"[1] we can finally find ourselves free of the untoward effects of the confusion and convoluted thinking of the human thought system, governed by ignorance of the truth. We honor God when we honor the truth of His established Creation and the Law of the Spirit of His One Life. We honor God when we know ourselves to be a part of this new creation in Christ, where all things are of God (good).

Continuing on in this chapter 5 of II Corinthians, we read that we, as this new creation, are to "know no man after the flesh, not even Jesus...but to see every man as this new creature, called Christ." Further we see that the purpose of our appearing as the Christ, is to "reconcile the world back to the truth, back to the true nature of God and to their position in Christ...by not imputing their trespasses unto them!" By not dealing with their sins and offenses at all...no judgment, no condemnation, no need to suffer to pay back a debt of sin...but instead by "not knowing them after the flesh." This means we are to deal with the world as all being in the One Life, manifesting the One Spirit. As we see this, they will respond and begin to feel it and know it themselves. How much better to reconcile the world to truth by knowing and declaring the truth of who they are than by consigning them to suffer for offences!

Chapter Seven

WHAT IS CHRIST?

Notice that the question here is not *who* is Christ, but *what* is Christ. The definition literally is the "visible expression of the invisible God."[1] Wherever God, or Love, or Life is revealed, manifested or declared...that is Christ, the visible expression of that which is invisible. That is why Jesus is called the Christ. He allowed the invisible God to express itself *as* his life. He understood, expressed and taught that this is the way of Life for all men. He called us children of Light and declared the richness of our inheritance in the Christ Life. He saw this everywhere and in everyone he met. He elevated man from his poor image of himself into the glorious liberty of the Son and Image of God.

Christ is not a person only but is wherever and whenever the Eternal beauty and perfection is revealed. For all things have their source and origin in the One Life.

Now that you understand the new covenant, you can understand why you are referred to as being "in Christ."

You are a manifestation of all the attributes and characteristics of the Eternal, as you accept this truth. This is what God sees. This is what Jesus saw when he healed the thousands and declared that sickness and suffering were not a necessary evil.

If you accept what Jesus came to declare, you will enjoy the benefits of it. If you do not accept this, you still are what you eternally are, but you will be like the man who desired to see a beautiful country and talked about it and read everything there was to read about it...and almost felt as though he had actually seen it...but never really did. There is a world of difference between thinking about something and actually experiencing it.

So we are told that we are "new creatures in Christ." We are told that all the old is passed away and all new has come. We are told that from now on everything is of God. This is not something that will happen...this is something that *has* happened. It is time to stop looking ahead, waiting for something to happen, but believe that it is present now and enter into that experience. This is the long desired "return of Jesus Christ" which will appear "to those who look for him...without sin unto salvation."[2] His appearing is in and through his body, which body you are!

How do we enter in? "Those who are *led by the Spirit of God* shall be called the sons of God."[3] Realizing that our life is not "our own" but that we have been sent here with a definite purpose is the beginning of "entering in." This will cause us to give up any extreme sense of personal responsibility for our bodies, and for the decisions we will need to make in our lives. We will have a sense of this life as being an expression of the One Life, and then as decisions come up, we will be able to pause and ask for counsel and wisdom and direction...and know that we will receive it. We will no longer be a personal possessor of many things, but a steward of all things. We will possess only the nature of God, which includes all things. The 44th chapter of Ezekiel reads, "*I am* their inheritance and *I am* their possession." Can you image such words being uttered by the voice of God! "*I am* their possession and *I am* their inheritance." That we belong to God is undisputed, but to know that the Life of God, with all its goodness and bounty and wisdom and clarity, harmony and health, *belongs to us!*

This is the development of the Christ consciousness. This is what it means to "be in Christ." To fully embrace this as *who and what* we are, takes a radical reliance on truth... and an absolute rejection of all that would appear contrary to it. To do this we must wait in silence with a heart full of desire to know truth from the mind and heart of God alone. For too long we have leaned upon the "knowledge" of man. Now we must begin to seek and to search out the hidden things of God and the truth of our oneness, in and as, the Christ of God. This comes by revelation and revelation comes by desire. And is freely given to all men.

SECTION FOUR

INTRODUCTION

PROBABLY THE MOST DIFFICULT to understand, this section dissects the man-made doctrines concerning the source and origin of evil, how it all started and where it all started. It examines what we have heard about evil being the true nature of all men. It discovers our current beliefs about the power of evil and then contrasts that with what we know about the nature of God, specifically His omnipotence (all power).

Here we look at the question of sin, of judgment and of the *innocence* of man's true and basic nature. And if innocent, then unworthy of punishment and not subject to the influence of evil.

Of all that I have understood and taught, the answers to these questions have caused some of the greatest reactions from religious, traditional theorists than any other. And having been where they are, I can certainly understand their discomfort.

Even so, I look forward with a confident heart to the

day when all honest seekers of truth will together embrace this. Because when the light of this understanding bursts forth into the hearts of mankind, we will be living in the "new heaven and new earth" that John wrote of. A place devoid of the suffering we now see all around us. This place has always been available to us, but as with anything else that has proven illusive and impossible to reach, we find we have been looking in the wrong direction to see it. Now we gladly join with those, whose passion for the truth and the courage to look again, have enabled them to find their way into this realm of existence.

CHAPTER ONE

OMNIPOTENCE VS.
THE POWER OF EVIL
EXAMINING THE ROOT OF EVIL

WHEN EXAMINING THE ROOT OF EVIL we must not only look at all aspects of human and religious thought, but the Divine Nature, as well. For God is the Creator of all and the only power source which truly exists.

This can be a very confusing subject because there have been many and contradictory theories as to the source of evil which have been advanced by mankind. There are the theorists who hold that physical causation is the root of physical manifestations. To those folks all disease has a physical cause. These are the theories which cause us to fear our environment, our genetics and our bodies. This way of seeing life keeps us bound to the law of chance and afraid of life in general. This mind-set must advance a reason for every sneeze! In this paradigm, the concept of a sovereign God watching over us, ordering our steps, being our protector and our very Life, is denied.

In enters religion to clear up this confusion. Yes, it says, God is sovereign and does order our every step, but because of our sinful nature and propensity to offend God, He will lead us into "testing" and trials. This will be for our own good, to correct, punish or redirect us.

That these "God ordained" testings and trials sometimes kills us, is a mystery. And that for all our tears and prayers of contrition, they sometimes persists relentlessly, is also a mystery. That this "needful suffering" is as vicious to the innocent babies and children as it is to the "sinful adults" is mind-boggling, pointing to a God who is heartless and beyond pleasing... one to be feared and therefore served out from fear. The idea of God as being Love is impossible to reconcile in this prevaling religious concept of a God who uses evil for an ultimate gain.

We have all heard that God created man in His image and likeness, therefore perfect and eternal. That would make man full of wisdom, understanding, knowledge and power. He would, by nature then, manifest all the goodness and intelligence of His Creator. He would not be subject to change, destruction or damage. However, layered upon this immutable fact of eternal existence, religion has man disobeying God, yielding to temptation and therefore losing his Divine Nature. This justifies God sending evil into the lives of His beloved man.

Still looking for the origin of evil, we are told that another aspect of God's creation also rebelled against Him and became His enemy. These angels set out to destroy all of God's creation, hence the eternal resistance of good and evil forces in the earth.

Sinking deeper into this quicksand of doctrine, we have no explanation as to how God could possibly create such creatures of potential rebellion and destruction. If it is true that "each seed reproduces after its own kind," then does this make God also rebellious and self-destructive?

So we have added to the whole mess the doctrine of self-will. Men and angels have their own will. But if every aspect of man is the expression and manifestation of only the Divine Mind, how could that mind rebel against itself?

At this point religion has now created atheists and agnostics...and who can blame them? Either the whole concept of God is a farce or man has it all wrong.

I have found in my search for clarity one thing for sure and that is that no man can teach us truth. It is something each one of us must search out for ourselves. If we want to get it right, we would be wise not to consult man, science or religion. We are comforted by this absolute truth..."You have no need that any man teach you for the Spirit of truth will lead and guide you into all truth."[1] Each one of us must learn from God alone. Only the Divine Mind can instruct us about itself.

We have all been "as sheep led to the slaughter," but we have allowed this to happen. It is so much easier to follow the doctrines of men than to search out the truth for oneself. But remember the words of our Maker, "This is Life Eternal, that they may *know* me and Jesus Christ whom I have sent."[2] To "know" means to become "one" with something, to be intimately acquainted with someone. This can only happen by a personal relationship that involves communication and time spent. So far, most have known *about* God, but there is a world of difference between knowing about someone and knowing them on a personal basis. To know and love someone is to know their heart, their thoughts, their motivating purpose, what drives them, and what they love. It is possible and desirable to know God to this degree. Jesus said the difference between a servant and a son is that the son knows what the father is doing and has become a vital part of that intention. This is the only way to break free of the cold, hard doctrines of men that serve only to divide mankind from one another, and cause people to flee from the arms of their Creator. It is this place in your heart which will allow you to hear the heart of God and know truth.

So what of this phenomenon called evil? Can what we have heard throughout the ages be challenged and can truth finally emerge? And how will that pure truth affect mankind in this never ending struggle between good and evil, wholeness and disease, peace and hate, abundant goodness and stark poverty?

Like much of humankind I spent most of the years of my life doing battle with evil wherever it might appear. Disease was the greatest of evils to me and I fought against it with every tool at my disposal, on every level. I began with all the aggressive medical means, and when that became too invasive and destructive, I moved on to alternative therapies. Although far superior in both wisdom and results, it still could not change the consciousness of the vulnerability to disease and destruction. By that I mean it could not keep one from fearing disease or remove the general expectation of the possibility of becoming sick. We were still victims of whatever might arise.

During all these experiences I prayed constantly for clarity and direction, mostly to understand the meaning of all this anguish and bondage to evil. I prayed to God, who I believed was a power greater than the power of evil, to intervene and overcome whatever was overcoming the people. Too often the prayers did not have the desired effect. So what was wrong? Where was I missing it?

Also the increasing number of people who needed deliverance from illnesses was astonishing and just kept on coming! There was no way to physically keep up with the need and demand. I wondered daily how Jesus managed to reach the multitudes who came to him each day.

Then came the idea of omnipotence. God is good and God is omnipotent. The word literally means, "one power." One power source. Since both good and evil cannot come from the same source, and God is good and the only Creator, then where does evil come from and from what does it derive its power? "Does a fountain send forth at the same place sweet water and bitter? Can the fig tree bear olive berries? So no fountain can both yield salt water and fresh."[3]

"I am the Lord, I am He. There is none else. I am the first and the last. I share my power with no one."[4]

We have made evil as powerful as good. Most have evil much more powerful than good. This makes two powers, sometimes in conflict with each other, but other times as co-workers to the same end. Some have God and the devil (d-evil) personally fighting, with mankind caught in the middle. Some have God and d-evil in one accord toward the same goal...our growth or correction. In this doctrine we have God using d-evil for His purposes. Some have d-evil as an enemy of God, some have it as a servant of God. Sufficient to say it is all very confusing and contradictory, as are all doctrines of men.

Remember we were told that the day we received, (absorbed, took in) the knowledge of both good and evil, we would open ourselves up to death. Disease and suffering is death. War and poverty is death. Death wears many faces. It is the opposite of life. Just as the word *evil* is *live* spelled backwards, so is any acceptance of evil as a power or force a backward way of looking at life that can only yield death.

If God recognized evil as a power, He then would be doing exactly what he told us not to do. He would be partaking of the knowledge of two opposite and warring powers.

If evil is a person, or a being, then it is created by God...and the nature of the thing created must reflect the creator Himself. This makes God both good and evil.

Now let us consider evil from an entirely different perspective. Rather than a person or a created entity...let us consider evil to be simply "darkness in our understanding," remembering that *all things which appear begin as thought.* Since the visible world is the result of the invisible world of thought and imagination...evil appearances result from places in our minds where we have not yet experienced truth and light, thereby allowing the darkness that rules our minds to create all sorts of imagined horror. (We have all as children entered a dark room and because of the fear of darkness (unknown) imagined all sorts of evil to be present in that place.)

Now shifting back to the ideas of religion, the true origin of evil is the darkness we perceive because of the images of a punishing, wrathful God and our subsequent worthiness to receive such suffering. This image of God creates the evil we fear!

As images of fear and abandonment by God, and unworthiness in His sight, rule our hearts and minds, we as a collective human consciousness begin to experience a keen sense of vulnerability to suffering.

We have become so accustomed to accepting the most intrusive, painful experiences in our lives and attributing it to the love of God. Religion has taught us to do this. We first accept the consequences of evil then declare that God knew that we needed the experience, therefore in Love sent it to us. We have done this for so long that we have been memorized into seeing horrible situations and seeing "a good reason for them to exist." We call evil an act of Love. Is it no wonder that we haven't a clue of what experiencing real Divine Love in our lives might mean?

I have a dear friend whose three year old daughter was killed in a car accident. She was in a coma for one year before she died. This experience tore into her mother heart in a way that nothing else could. It shredded the heart of the father as well. It tore into the grandparents sensibililities until they still cannot speak of the child. Now the mother has said from the time she first told me the story that God used this to soften her heart and break through the proverbial hardness of the human heart.

Now here is my question. Who created her heart hard, only to, at a later date, need to send pain to recreate it again? Who said she needed the pain? Religion says that. So she has for years accepted this evil as having a "good and necessary cause," therefore, as being good. She has believed that this was the "love of God" towards her...confusing stark suffering with love, as does all religious notions such as this. Until we cease attempting to find a "religious and reasonable cause" for tragedies, and call them what they really are, which is the result of believing in a power of evil... we will continue to experience them. I have heard this same line of reasoning about evil, suffering and the love of God for forty years now and it is time that someone spoke up and defined and defended Love! Until we do this we will continue to accept evil and call it good!

Consider the word devil as simply *believing in evil*, in two opposing powers, *therefore opening ourselves to the experience of that which we hold in thought.*

Using the word "we," which is referring again to the collective human consciousness... we have not only allowed the thought of evil, we have built a shrine to the power of evil, fearing its effects much more than the power of God (good) in our lives.

Is darkness a power, or is it simply the absence of light...light being the power or energy source?

Is cold a power, or is it simply the absence of heat...heat being the power or energy source?

Are accidents a power or is it simply the lack of seeing only Divine Order and Harmony ruling its creation?

Is dis-ease a power, or is it simply believing in the absence of order and intelligence within the body...Divine Order and Infinite Intelligence being the power or energy source?

Is evil a power, or simply a belief in the absence of good...God being the only power or energy source?

And if evil is not a power, then from where does it derive its destructive nature? If not from our belief in its supposed power, our educated fear of it? Can we realize that if it is not a power, then it cannot be aggressive...it cannot hurt or harm?

Then why do we feel the effects of it?

Because we do not see God as being the only power.

And we do not see God as being only good!

So we give the suggestions of evil, as they appear in our lives, the place and space that belongs only to God.

The moment that we see the goodness and benevolence
of God as being greater than the evil that is presenting itself,
that is the moment evil will disappear.

Just as the moment we turn on the light, darkness disappears.

When speaking of the final fall of evil in the earth, Isaiah says in the 14th chapter, "How are thou cut to the ground, which did weaken the nations. For thou said in thine heart, I will ascend above the heights of the clouds: I will be like the Most High God. Yet thou shall be brought down to hell. They that see thee shall narrowly look upon thee saying, 'Is *this* what made the world to be as a wilderness and destroyed the cities?'"

In that day shall evil appear as the 'nothing' that it really is.

Evil is a thought. A thought which takes on the form of a substance. And just like any other thought that we do not wish to experience, we can learn the simplicity of dismissing it from our mind. *If we could stop worrying so much about ridding ourselves of the "appearance" that the thought produced, and go directly to the root (which is always thought)...we would see how readily and thoroughly we can eliminate evil and its effects from our lives.

Evil is a bully that will scatter and flee as a cockroach when the light is turned on. It is as nothing. The day will come when we will marvel at the attention we gave to it.

But until we see the all-ness, the goodness, and the only power as belonging to God...and therefore to us, as His image in the earth... we will yet tremble at the appearance of evil, giving it the only power it can possibly have.

CHAPTER TWO

COULD IT BE?

COULD IT BE THAT IF WE ACTUALLY...

• Acknowledged God as the only power;

• Acknowledged that power as only good;

• Denied the dichotomy of both good and evil as a legitimate human experience;

• Denied a punishing God and actually believed that the "goodness of God would lead all men to repentance;" (to a change in understanding and direction)

• Learned to expect only good from God, from others, from life, from ourselves;

• Determined to fill our hearts and thoughts and our expectations with only goodness;

• Learned that evil is only a *thought externalized*, and as such, habitually 'send it away" from us, from everyone (this is the true definition of forgiveness, 'to send away').

Could it be then that evil would cease to exist?

We are told in the Bible that evil will one day cease to exist. We all look forward to the "new heaven and new earth"[1] when this will actually happen. This would be the answer to the prayer that Jesus taught which said, "Thy will be done here on earth just as it is in heaven." Instead of believing that overcoming evil with force will finally put it to rest? We are told by Jesus to "resist not evil,"[2] telling us that the more we resist it the more power we are giving to it and the more it will appear in our lives.

The greatest challenge we have at the clinic daily, hourly, is to keep the *expectation of good* "alive and active" in the minds and hearts of the patients. We have found that when they hold to the *dread of evil*...the power of the disease...they do not recover.

If they can release that fear and dread, experiencing instead the expectation of goodness, of Life appearing...they always recover.

We do it first by believing it ourselves, and then by teaching the omnipotence and goodness of God. As long as this is the prevailing thought, all goes well. But heaven help us when darkness is allowed to enter their hearts once again.

So we talk to them about becoming, "watchmen on the wall." Being vigilant about their thoughts, the company they keep, where they go and what they listen to, in order to protect their thoughts and expectations. We dread their going back to hear reports from the medical community as it so often proves to paralyze them back into fear, and immediately symptoms regain their foothold. Remember everything is first "thought."

This story is one of thousands...but it remains with

me today, so I will share it with you. It illustrates the power of evil imaginations:

Karla was from west Texas and she had a brain tumor. Actually she had one tumor in her lung and several in her brain. When I met her she was staggering down the hallway to my office, leaning on a walker for support. She had recently undergone brain surgery to reduce the size of the largest tumor and had a wig on her head, but it was perched up there crooked. She had undergone at least two craniotomies (brain surgeries) to scoop out the tumors, but of course, they continued to return. Karla was confused, disoriented and hostile. But her family adored her and assured me that their mom never had a "mean moment" in her life.

She moved to San Antonio, with her sister to care for her, and began the program. Within weeks the tumors began to "melt down" and appeared as a black substance in her mouth. It was pretty nasty for her, but it eventually stopped happening. Although we usually ask for four months of treatment before going back for tests, her husband took her in **for** repeat tests in two months. There was not one tumor left on the MRI, not even in the lung!

Karla's attitude had become completely different. She was pleasant and coherent and endearing to every one of us. I especially loved her. It was during this time that my sister was so sick and I was traveling to California almost weekly until she eventually passed away. Every morning when I came to the clinic I would find a card from Karla on my desk with a sweet note inside to encourage me. It was easy to see why her family loved her so much.

Karla remained well and doing great for several months. She moved back home to west Texas and just drove to us for check ups every week. But one day she received a call either from her son, or about her son, I'm not sure. The content of the call was devastating to her. He was evidently involved in something that saddened her to the point of collapse. Less than a month later the tumors were back and soon found to have spread. She never recovered from the image of evil that overcame her soul that day.

Now is this how evil appears? Is this how it derives it power?

So many thousands of sick folks have testified that their illness began right after a severe emotional response, a catastrophic fear or disappointment, something that weakened their usual defense.

We know the devastation that the endocrine system experiences during such an emotional event. We know what havoc the metabolism endures. Many folks say that they gained uncontrollable weight during or right after such an event of tragedy in their lives.

This is why it is so important for us to quickly deny the power of evil when it appears and acknowledge the omnipotence of only good (God).

There is a verse I quote a lot from Psalms which says, "I would rather be a doorkeeper in the house of God than to sit at a banquet table with fools."[3] The "house of God" is our consciousness...our minds...what we know and believe and therefore experience. Otherwise known as our souls. To be a "doorkeeper" is one who watches what comes into thought and keeps unwanted thoughts and suggestions of evil out. Here, a "fool" is one who allows the events that appear to enter indiscriminately and remain, as though they had a legitimate right to rule our lives!

This is why it is so important for us to really understand the true nature of God and to resist the doctrines of men. If we believe the lies and the confusion we have heard about God, we will not know that whatever is appearing *has no right to exist*, and that we have the power and right and authority to send it away! If we believe, for instance, that God is "using this event for our good"...then that undermines our ability to deal with it...and we just let it remain, to "steal, to kill and to destroy."[4]

Just a few years ago a lady came to our weekly meetings where I spoke of these truths. I was teaching specifically that disease is an intruder. It is not sent by God and has no authority or purpose to exist. Since we are created in the image of God, we have the authority to deny its existence.

One night this dear lady must have really heard it. She had suffered for 11 years with a condition known as interstitial cystitis. To reduce this to common terms, she had a chronically inflamed urinary bladder that made her urinate nearly constantly and burned like fire, day and night. The only medical treatment for this is to remove the bladder surgically and wear bags to catch the urine flow for the rest of her life. You can see why she continued to suffer for so long. Not too many people would consent to that very readily.

This one particular night, during the throws of a severely painful attack, she decided to become the master of the situation and no longer the slave of her own body! So she played a game. "Knock, knock." "Who's there?" "Pain, and I have come to make your night and your life miserable." "Who invited you?" she demanded. "I never invited you. Go away! You are not welcome. I do not give my consent for you to remain!"

Much to her amazement the pain left! She told us that she had to repeat that scenario four times that night before it finally left for good. I asked her if it ever reappeared and she said, "Four times. Each time after a stressful day. But each time I sent it away and it finally never came back."

After 11 years of such intense suffering, she was finally free, just by understanding who she was and where she came from. Just by learning her true identity and finding the true nature of God... and therefore, the illegitimacy of evil to appear.

It is true that to get to this understanding, we must leave behind the mainstream of human thought. Sometimes it feels like we're swimming upstream, when everyone else is floating with the current of popular human belief. But the cost has been too great to continue downstream. And the rewards for our efforts are too abundant to deny.

This understanding makes it clear that all intelligence, strength, form, beauty, harmony, immutable order, function, procreation, motion, direction, and purpose for existence, has its origin and continued presence in the mind of the only Creator, God the Eternal Good.

Simply put, *Life comes from the Creator only, and not*

from that which has been created. Our bodies cannot give us life, and unless we unknowingly allow it, our bodies cannot take life away. Other people cannot give us happiness, and unless we allow it, they cannot take it away either. Career opportunities cannot give us prosperity, and unless we allow it, they cannot take anything away from us either.

God is sovereign. God is omnipotent. And God is good. That truly is all we really need.

CHAPTER THREE

WHAT IS SIN?

SIN IS NOT TRANSGRESSION OF THE LAW. That is called transgression. In the Old Testament there was a sacrifice for sin and a sacrifice for transgressions, signifying that these are two separate things.

Sin is entertaining a "sense of separation from God." It is a consciousness, a nature...not an action. The sin consciousness is that which is blind to the true nature of God and man, as he is created. It is the root and the beginning of evil.

It started with the "knowledge of good and evil," that old dichotomy of thought that caused us to perceive something other than Life. The knowledge that caused us to forget who we were, and why we were sent. The knowledge that caused us to forget who formed us and in what nature we were created.

All this caused a sense of separation from God, from Life,

from Mercy, from Goodness, from realizing that we are eternal beings...never starting, never ending.

So the whole human thought...the whole human consciousness is called sin. Sin is a nature, a consciousness...not a transgression of the law. *Transgressions occur because we are dwelling in this sin nature.* So far, collectively, we have seen ourselves out from this sin consciousness, because we have been taught to see this way.

The conscious awareness of a sin nature must be *replaced* with another, higher awareness of being. *True* forgiveness is not covering a particular offense, or releasing someone from an injury done, but actually *replacing the thought* (belief) that caused the offense with another, higher thought. And that can only come by the arrival of a new understanding.

The sin consciousness is a consciousness of inferiority and unworthiness in the sight of God. It comes from a sense of separation from both the nature and mind of God. Entering into the Christ consciousness, accepting that nature as our nature, living out from that understanding with a confident rejoicing...this is the only way of escape.

Simply dealing with individual offenses is like cutting off diseased branches and leaving the cause of the disease still intact within the tree, only to have it appear again at a later time. This is no different than dealing with individual diseases, leaving intact the consciousness that accepted the experience as valid, although unwanted, allowing it to appear.

Can you see how the harsh judgment of man, and religion in particular, convincing us that we are less than what we really are? Do you see that only by a revelation of the truth of our eternal, intact, present and permanent perfection by the Spirit of Life, as our life, will we ever be able to see and know only Life again...never again empowering darkness and evil?

CHAPTER FOUR

THE JUDGMENT OF GOD IS MERCY

*"The mercy of God is from everlasting
to everlasting...it fails not."*[1]

If there is one continuing theme throughout the scriptures it is that of mercy.

The Old Testament Israelites knew little about the concept of mercy. Their understanding of God was fearful and harsh. His judgments were swift and exacting.

This was their vision of God, with one exception...God lived in a place called the Mercy Seat. This was located in the innermost room of the tabernacle that Moses erected, known as the Tabernacle in the Wilderness. The Mercy seat *covered* the Arc of the Covenant which contain among other things, the Ten Commandments. Since it was located *above the laws and statutes,* God was telling them that *mercy excelled above the just demands of the law.* But they did not understand that then and rarely do we understand it even now.

King David wrote at length that the heart of God was mercy. He seemed to understand the nature of God far and away beyond the rest of the people. Right in the midst of the era of the blood sacrifices to atone for the transgressions of the law, he made this startling discovery when he said, "Sacrifices and offerings for sin you do not require. My ear hast thou opened."[2] David came to realize that God was much more interested in a personal relationship with His creation, one that heard His voice and delighted to respond to Him, than the repetitive oblations for sin.

David also wrote that God *required mercy*...that we *accept* mercy and that we *show* mercy...rather than live the most devoted and sacrificial life possible.

Much later Jesus brought the concept of mercy to a very blind and confused people. When a woman was caught in adultery, a crime worthy of death, Jesus pricked their consciences with the words, "Let him who has never sinned cast the first stone." He demonstrated the heart of God by showing her mercy, forgoing the judgment required by the law.

Instead of embracing such a warm and beautiful concept, instead of becoming overwhelmed with gratitude for such a liberating understanding of the true nature of God...the religious leaders became incensed with this man. Who did he think he was coming and changing everything they knew to be true? What about their laws? What about the necessity for suffering to pay back the debt of sin?

Worse yet, what would become of mankind if they never had to face God's judgment? Wouldn't that be a "license to continue sinning?"

And what about all those required "blood sacrifices?" What then are they all about?

They hated Jesus for the turmoil and confusion he was causing. He was shaking their most cherished foundations and threatening everything they knew. A few of the religious leaders, like Nicodemus, actually got it...but most did not.

At one point while they were grilling him about this "new doctrine," he boldly repeated the words of David from long ago and declared, *"I will have mercy and not sacrifice, go and learn what that means!"*[3]

Later still, James wrote these profound words, *"Mercy rejoices against judgment."*[4] Mercy is from a higher atmosphere of thought. Mercy excels over judgment. It is more to be desired than judgment. Mercy *is* the judgment of God![5]

Now what is this thing called mercy? Mercy is not compassion. Compassion is compassion. Mercy is not forgiveness. Forgiveness is forgiveness.

Mercy is the ability to see through and beyond that which appears, to that which is eternal and never changes.

Mercy is how God always sees His creation. When mercy touches our heart...it changes us forever. We are never the same. We are healed. Our lives are corrected. All things become new. We are then able to see who we really are and why we are called "new creatures in Christ." Simply because we were made that way!

Every time we chose to see someone as they are created, in the beauty and excellence of their Creator, instead of holding on to what we are seeing visibly...we have just healed them. The Christ of their being is stirred and arises, "with healing in his wings."

Always God sees us as we truly are, and *as we are able to perceive it,* we are healed. We are made aware of our holiness and completeness. A whole new vision of ourselves dawns upon our hearts and all impulse to sin is removed. Mercy is how 'one conscious awareness' is replaced with another...the human consciousness of sin and suffering, is replaced with the Divine consciousness of holiness and innocence.

Judgment can never do that! Judgment is a constant reminder of our sins and failures. Judgment might keep us in line for awhile, but it can never change us. It can never heal us. It can never cause our true nature to be revealed to us.

Judgment governs by fear. Mercy governs by truth and Love!

We have come from the Mind of God to reveal to man his true nature, just as Jesus came to reveal to us our true nature. "As my Father sent me, so send I you."[6] This is the message of the Christ. There is one way that this is done and only one way. God does it for us, and we must do it for others. That is to deal with mankind according to mercy.

We must learn to see beyond the visible offenses. To learn to see beyond the diseased beliefs and experiences. To learn to see beyond the limitations man imposes upon himself. To learn to see that which never changes.

This is a prerequisite to true forgiveness. Forgiveness

means "to send away." True forgiveness is to see through the eyes of mercy to the real man created in and as the likeness of God. To cease seeing the offense of the man and to send it away from him. *We separate the offense from the offender* and we send the offense away...by not "imputing" the offense to him. By not "attributing it to his account."

This is not the way forgiveness has been defined to us. We think that we are to first *acknowledge* the offense, then out of the kindness of the heart, forgive someone his injury against us. That is nice to keep human relations in harmony, but it does not heal the man.

It does not enable him to be free of the belief that is causing him to offend. Only by NOT seeing the offense as part of his nature and separating him from it, can we send it away and heal him.

David said, "Blessed is the man whom the Lord does not impute iniquity."[7]

In other words, blessed is the one who realizes that God sees beyond the offense into the real man. Blessed is the one who knows that God separates the man from the offense, not assigning it to an account, but sending it away!

This is a far cry from the God "who sees all and writes it in His book to settle the score in an eternal hell."

This is exactly how we are healed. This is exactly how we are to heal others from their offenses, from attitudes of the heart, *from disease*, from limitations...from everything and anything plaguing mankind.

If we try to do this by our own efforts, by repeating words and phrases shallow to the ones needing mercy...we will not see the healings that we desire. But if we *yield ourselves to the Heart of Mercy Itself,* Mercy will see *for us* what we could not see by our own ability.

A great power is released when Mercy is truly in the midst of us. All the power of the Eternal, endless Life.

Of all the teachings here that conflict with the religious doctrine of the day, this is the one that seems to excite more anger and fury than the rest. Pastors and teachers of the scriptures return my words of mercy with the "needful justice of God." They believe that man's justice and God's justice are one and the same. Man punishes man for offenses; that is the law of sowing and reaping. But God's definition of justice is mercy, not judgment!

Too many religious leaders cling to the doctrine of eternal punishment for all those who do not qualify for heaven. They misunderstand the nature of God and they have missed the entire message of mercy that Jesus came to reveal to us. I remember a woman once preached, "If God does not punish and destroy San Francisco, then He needs to apologize to Sodom and Gomorrah!" This is a propensity for self-righteousness that knows no bounds! No wonder those who hold to this type of doctrine suffer the same diseases and divorces and destruction as the rest of the "heathen" world! No wonder that when they need and look for mercy, it escapes them as well.

Lest anyone be confused here, I am not turning a blind eye to evil and the terribleness of the sin nature or sin consciousness. I am not advocating a "namby pamby, live and let live, anything goes, if it feels good do it" philosophy. We are sent to *heal* whenever evil rears its ugly head. We are sent, not to judge the individual by what we see or hear, but to "judge righteously," To judge according to the true nature of the individual. This is mercy and this will heal.

Unrighteous judgment is evil. Turning a blind eye, so as to be politically correct and not judge anyone, is equally as evil. We are sent to heal and this is the way it is to be done.

Mercy is the Divine Life declaring, "I am here and I never change, *I am not a reactive God.* I do not react to human beliefs, human fears, human limitations, human creations of thought or human error. I am constant with what I know and what I see. I see right through it all. I see *myself* in all that I have formed." This is how Jesus healed, this is how we are healed and this is how we are to heal others.

II Samuel said, "To the merciful, I will appear merciful."

Jesus said, "Blessed are the merciful, for they shall obtain mercy."[8]

We are transformed by mercy, but it will avail us nothing unless we take up the Divine purpose for our existence, and learn to see through the heart of mercy to transform others.

If we judge and do not see present perfection in all God's creation, then when we need it ourselves, we will not be able to see it there either...or receive it.

CHAPTER FIVE

RETURN TO INNOCENCE

INNOCENCE DOES NOT MEAN IGNORANCE, but rather it means not tainted with evil or guilt. It means having a conscience utterly devoid of contamination from a sense of separation from the total acceptance of God.

No matter where you are or what your history might be, God is never against you. Because the darkness that may be influencing you...that which seeks to destroy you... is *not coming from you!* It may look like it. It may feel like it. You may be acting like it. But no evil can arise from within you. You are created in the image of God! And as soon as you know this *you will cease to act out from evil's suggestions.*

Until you realize your true nature, you can be influenced by the evil thoughts of the human consciousness, which is devoid of the Spirit of God. But those thoughts do not come from you. You are "hid with Christ in God." *You are existing as Eternal Life's manifestation of Itself.*

Until the full reality of this is understood, you will

continue to beg and plead for help from God because your vision of God will be *coming from your own sense of failure* and the fearful expectation of the punishment and wrath of God. But you must not seek to overcome God's *reluctance* to intervene, by begging and pleading, for there *is no reluctance*! There can be no reluctance or God would not be good. God would not be Love. God would not be immutable.

If your children were in trouble, even of their own making, and they turned to you for help and you were absolutely able to help them, would you withhold your help? Maybe some would. But that is only because some folks seem to be far away from knowing the heart of Mercy. Most everyone would answer, "Yes!"

Know this then...that your demonstration of love toward your children comes from the Love of God residing within your heart. That is how He loves you. So if there seems to be any hesitation in the help appearing, that hesitation is not coming from God, but from our inability to *receive*. The human sense of guilt, coupled with the distorted image of a wrathful God, is the cause of the lack of *receptivity*.

You must *feel* innocent and you must *feel* loved before you can receive a healing or anything from God. That is because it is your own *sense of guilt and unworthiness* that caused the problem to start with. To experience anything from the realm of absolute goodness, you must enter the mind and heart of God. You must leave behind what the human consciousness declares and know what God is.

This is why it is so important for us to know the truth.

We are not the source of evil or disease, although it may appear to us that we are. We must know the truth about man's true nature, despite the appearance... and then separate ourselves from this strange appearance of suffering or evil.

We are not what is appearing. We are God's image and reflection of Himself in every case. It honors God for us to know and stand in this truth. It dishonors God for us to deny it. That is false humility.

To know this is the beginning of returning to innocence in our minds and heart.

It is not good enough for us to simply say the words. We must *pray* the words. We must desire for God to reveal the truth to our hearts. This is a prayer that is quickly answered every time it is uttered!

One of my favorite stories in the Bible is that of the prophet, Daniel. At the time, Daniel, along with all the Israelites, had been taken into captivity by the nation of Babylon. This is very significant to us remembering that the word Babylon means "the confusion of many voices." This is our present day circumstance. We also are taken into captivity by so many different voices, all them declaring that they are the one we should listen to and live our lives according to their particular belief system.

We have the 'religious Babylon' that declares we are meant to suffer, that we are poor and wretched and altogether sinful, needing to suffer to cleanse us from our many transgressions. This distortion of truth also declares that we belong to a God who watches us to mark in His book when we miss the proverbial mark! Living out from this Babylonian ideology, we can't do anything *but* miss the mark. The mark keeps moving!

We have the god of science, which declares that we are nothing more than matter, with our beginnings as a DNA molecule. This consigns us to living under the law of chance and probability, enduring whatever cards that are dealt us. The fear and uncertainty that this Babylonian nonsense produces is enough to cause our minds and bodies to end up dis-eased, as predicted! Our minds and bodies were not created to live under such confusion and uncertainty. This is how fear creates the object that is feared!

Being "taken into captivity" to any of these thoughts causes us to be lulled into a state of stupor, a non-thinking existence that will accept whatever comes as either being "the cards dealt" or the "will of god." Not realizing that a change in conscious understanding will correct whatever the present circumstance.

So this was where Daniel found himself, a captive to the confusion of many voices. When he refused to bend to the demands of those "gods," he was consigned to the den of lions. For us, this den of lions could be anything that we might be presently facing; a disease, a destruction of any sort...whatever appears as less than the goodness and abundance and glory of God in our life.

The interesting thing here is that when the king came to the mouth of the den early the next morning to see how chewed up Daniel really got, he was greeted with these words from a very alive Daniel... "God sent his angels to shut the mouths of the lions so that no hurt was found on me *in that innocence was found in me!*"[1]

There it is! Because Daniel knew that God saw innocence in him, he was spared the horrible ordeal. Daniel knew this because he knew *both the nature of God and the truth of man created in His image.* He did not let that which appeared, no matter how convincing it might have been, distract him from this absolute truth. He maintained his innocence. *Not because he believed that he earned it.* Not because of anything having to do with him at all. But because he knew what was true and what was false. He did not judge according to appearances, but according to the truth. It is not surprising then to learn that the name Daniel means "the righteous judgment of God!"

To really see yourself innocent, you must see *all* of God's creation as innocent also. Remember that everything formed came from the same One Life, with all the attributes and nature of that One Life.

There are many who teach the "we they" doctrine. "We are righteous, they are not. We are saved, they are not. We are holy and beloved, they are not. We chose God, they did not." People who embrace this doctrine have fallen into the teachings of men and confused them with the teachings of God.

The truth is that Jesus said, "You have not chosen me, but I have chosen you."[2] We, each one, have been sent that a specific purpose may be fulfilled. It is this very purpose that *finds us!*

Unless we embrace all of creation under the absolute innocence of the nature of God...we will never be able to embrace it for ourselves. For God said, "Ye are the true light that cometh into the world." He said that He was the light of *all men*. He said that *all men have received the fullness of God!*[3]

I remember a man who came to my office in a terminal state of illness with multiple bone fractures from cancer. He had already lost over 70 pounds and looked like walking death.

He had lived his life in a very self-serving manner. He was a ruthless business man who did not seek the good of anyone but his own, at the expense of everyone in his life. He had five wives and several children, none of whom he raised. He was also an alcoholic.

The day came when I believed he was ready to hear the truth of who he really was and the nature of the goodness of God. I wasn't too sure if he might not just walk out when I started to talk, but I figured that to not say anything would be certain death.

I was surprised and delighted that he embraced the words with tears and a desire to do whatever he needed to do. I told him that he must see everyone else in his life, in the world for that matter, through the same eyes that God saw him. So he made a list of everyone he had previously hated and the list was pages long. He also made a list of those to whom he had been hurtful, and that also was pages long. He set out to contact everyone on those lists.

He apologized to all of them. He spoke kind words to

those who he had misjudged, which was everyone! In general he attempted to bridge the gaps and repair the damage done throughout his life. It took months but he hung on. He once said that this was the happiest that he ever felt in his life. He said that if he died it would be okay because he finally understood why he was here and how he was supposed to live. But he didn't die. Four months later all the cancer was gone and all the bones were healed. You couldn't even tell which bones had been broken!

What happened? *As he declared the goodness and innocence of others, he began to realize it for himself.* All guilt and condemnation had vanished. For the first time since he arrived into this mortal existence, he felt his Divine Nature emerge. He was lifted up into an atmosphere of thought that only knew health and joy and abundant goodness. This was a place where dis-ease simply could not exist.

Simply put, if you cannot forgive yourself, it is because you cannot forgive another. If you cannot see goodness in yourself, it is because you are not seeing it in others. If you cannot realize innocence in yourself, it is because you do not see others as pure and innocent and altogether good.

This is why those who profess religion become just as sick as those who do not. Religion is not an insurance policy against sickness and confusion in our lives, *but knowing the truth* of God and man *is.*

SECTION FIVE

CHAPTER ONE

THE RHYTHM OF LIFE

THERE IS A "RHYTHM OF LIFE" that flows throughout all of creation, indeed throughout all infinity. It is a constant pulsation of life that all things formed responds to, from the stars to the tiniest insect. You feel this rhythm with every beat of your heart. All creation feels it and lives by it.

You cannot see this rhythm, but then you cannot see air either. You cannot see the wind, but you can feel the effects of its presence. Just like air, we depend upon it for our entire being. This rhythm is the Presence that formed all that we see and are, and this is the Presence that holds it all together in perfect order.

This perpetual rhythm flows whether we are realizing it or not. It remains constant no matter what else might be going on. It is not subject to the opinions or beliefs of mankind, changeable and unsubstantial as they are. It is constant, perpetual, eternal, immutable (unchangeable). *It responds to its own intelligent order only.* And wherever it is, Life and beauty, perfection and goodness, and absolute order prevails.

We realize this rhythm as we look out upon the stars of our galaxy, as we see the order of the planets and the orbits they effortlessly follow. We see the seasons as they come and go, revealing to us the necessity of periods of time to lie dormant (winter), to withdraw in quietness and stillness to replenish our thoughts and clear our hearts of the foolishness and clamor of the human consciousness, only to enjoy newness of Life (spring) as it emerges out from those times of reflection. These are ways that the infinite Intelligence, that we call God, speaks to us to impart wisdom and understanding that eventually leads us to know Who and What He is and what our relationship is to that Being.

Reflecting still upon this current of Life or 'rhythm,' consider the animals, each one following certain patterns of activity depending upon its species. Who directs the squirrel to hide nuts for the oncoming winter? Who determines the various seasons of birthing and gives wisdom to the mother in caring for her young? What unseen, but definite influence directs, maintains and sustains all things created, from the creatures to the plants and trees? "He opens His hand and satisfies the desire of every living thing."[1]

There is a rhythm of Life, a current of 'energy,' intelligent and wise, constant and perpetual that formed all that is visible, that fills all things, determines the existence of all, and directs the activity of all. *It is the Life and breath of all that it has formed.* It is also referred to as the Spirit of the Life of all things.

Interestingly, the root word for 'breath' is the same root

word for 'spirit' and 'air'...all being 'pneumo'. Just as the air fills all space, so does this Spirit of Life fill all space and place. It knows no vacuum. Where ever there is space provided, it will instantly fill it. So we read that "We live and move and have our being in this rhythm/Spirit of Life." As does all of creation.

God is not separate from that which He has created!

As we said earlier, we come to understand the nature of this Life flow (God) by that which It has made. Creation declares its Creator!

So throughout this vast expanse of visible creation we begin to know and feel and realize the constant Presence of this rhythm of all Life. In moments of quietness and stillness we can feel ourselves being in the midst of it, being carried by the flow of it. Soon it becomes more real to us than that which we see. We know that we are truly alive and that it is alive as it flows through us, bringing Life to every cell, every organ, every system, every nook and cranny and crevice of our bodies, our minds, our thoughts and emotions, establishing and maintaining order throughout our entire lives.

• No more do we look to our bodies to bring Life and health to us, for we now realize that our bodies merely *respond* to the Presence of the rhythm of eternal, infinite Life.

• No more do we make the mistake of thinking that anything made (created) has the ability to live out from itself, separate and independent of the Spirit of Life that formed it.

• No more do we depend upon the body for our strength, our health, our well-being.

Now we look to the Life of all things, the Life of *us*. Now we look to the *rhythm*, the Presence of Life itself and that now becomes the *source of our Life and all the desired goodness in it*.

Why is this important? How does this, in and of itself change anything? How does it make us more secure in our health, our safety, our lives?

All I knew, or thought I knew, about life and death was believing that we were responsible for it all. I had been trained as an ICU nurse; I had spent much of my life running around frantically trying to fix what was broken, right what was wrong and in general feeling very responsible for the outcome of it all. In my world the life of the body was very fragile, apt to come apart at any moment, often with no warning at all. Sound familiar?

Each organ, each system and each cell was responsible to maintain its own order and do what was right. If it didn't... and we never really thought that it would or could...then we were the ones who needed to fix it. Most of the "medical thought" today is either running around frantically, captivated by this illusion of feeling very responsible...or floating in a fog of apathy, having long ago realized that we can't fix a thing.

This is called human intervention and the entire medical world exists and functions within this thought. Actually the entire "world thought" is an expression of this belief. Within this atmosphere of thought we have no trust, no confidence and no understanding of what life is at all.

For years I lived in this convoluted and disordered

thought. Weren't we supposed to fix what was wrong? Weren't we supposed to fear that which could hurt? Wasn't life full of threats that we needed to concern ourselves with in order to avoid them when possible? How could one possibly trust life when life obviously could not be trusted at all?

For a long time it was so very frustrating for me. I couldn't grasp it and I couldn't let it go. I found myself crying from the frustration and confusion of my thoughts.

It was this frame of thought which brought me to the experience of the knowledge, and more importantly, *the feeling of Life*. This was an *eternal truth*, aching to reveal itself to me.

☙

One night, while sound asleep from the exhaustion of the events of the previous day, Life broke through the mist and maze of my confusion. *Life...* with all of its glory and brilliance, clarity and purity... with all of its goodness and perfection, burst forth with these words,

"There is only ONE LIFE. I AM that Life. Everything exists as a manifestation of that Life. Everyone exists as a manifestation of that Life."

The whole experience was electrifying. I bolted upright in my bed.

Suddenly I was able to *see* the Life of everything. Not just the visible, but the Life of it all. I saw that this Life was the governing Presence, as it filled all form and gave beauty and order to everything. I saw that God was not separate from anything, needing to be prayed to in order to fix anything, but was actually the Life of everything already!

For months this awareness stayed with me. It was effortless and more 'real' to me than anything I had previously believed. God was the Life of all and all was the manifestation of that one Life.

Needless to say, my entire thought system, my entire belief system took an immediate and radical shift. Pieces of the proverbial puzzle began to fall into place. I began to understand things that I had read in my Bible, which up until then had made no sense to me at all.

The thing that was most important to me was that now I understood how it was that Jesus healed all those sick and suffering folks. He always saw Life, not the images of sick, pathetic humans that came to him for help. He saw what never changes... what God, the Life of all things, made and maintains. He chose to see beyond what was believed into the heart of what cannot be altered. He saw Life... everywhere, in everything. He traveled through this human experience knowing what no one else at the time knew. He came to teach this to us. *You see nothing needed to be fixed...only seen correctly.* What we call a healing was what Jesus saw as ever-present reality.

Of course Jesus saw with his eyes what everyone else saw, but definitely not with his heart. In other words, *he never agreed to it, never gave his consent to it.* How come? Because He knew something infinitely more real than imperfection and affliction. He knew that Life was the real issue here and not what we saw, experienced or believed. It begs the question, "Do we experience these things because we first believe that our lives are fragile and subject to such afflictions? And is it these very beliefs that allow such things to appear? And if so, how are these beliefs corrected? With what eyes are we able to see the Life of us that is whole and perfect, beautiful and eternal?"

Healings are not miracles, but the *natural consequence* of knowing life as it truly is. Healings are not corrections that appear, but simply the removal of one thought and the replacement with another. Even though we do not always see the perfect, it is always present. It is only the false image of thought which needs to be replaced with the true.

We need to realize that Life is not what we are *doing*, but the Presence of an un- interruptible rhythm, an unseen, invisible Spiritual Presence, who is revealing itself as, and through, all that it has made. We then can allow it to reveal itself to us... and eventually as us. Then there truly will appear the Oneness of God and man, and the prayer of Jesus will be fulfilled, "That they may be one as we are one, we in them and they in us..."[2] One! Perfect God, perfect Life flowing in perfect rhythm, establishing and maintaining perfect order everywhere it *is seen and acknowledged.*

Being a Bible student, I began to remember stories and events, words and truths, here and there that finally made sense to me. Some of these I will share with you now.

In the second book of the Kings, we meet a dynamic prophet named Elijah. During his ministry he mentors a young aspiring prophet named Elisha. Never before had there been documented such miracles and wonders as Elijah per-formed. So when it came time for him to return to the Spirit which sent him, he asked his young friend what he would like Elijah to do for him before he left. Elisha answered that he would like "a double portion of your Spirit to rest upon me." He wanted to continue the same works that his master had done. He wanted to truly follow in his footsteps. After a thoughtful moment Elijah answered him. "If you are able to *see* me *after I am taken from you*, it shall be done unto you."[3]

In order to see Elijah after he was gone, he would need to be able to *see* with the eyes of his heart. He needed to *see* beyond what was visible... into the eternal truth of God. Namely, *that God is the Life of men and that Life never ceases to exist. When that Life is known and realized, then the ever- present perfection and beauty of it will be what appears to men.* Evidently Elisha was able to see what Elijah saw during his time here, because he continued in his master's work performing the same works that he did.

Later in the account of the book of John, Jesus said to his followers, "Greater works than these shall *you* do, after I am gone to my Father."[4] Just prior to this he was telling them that his time here was finished, but even though they would not *see* him, yet they would soon *be able* to *see* him. This could be rather confusing unless you begin to realize that he is speaking of the seeing that is done with the heart because of an enlightened understanding. And what is that understanding? Namely that He, the Christ, is the Life of all men... all creation in fact. And as soon as you are able to see that clearly, and no longer see only as man sees... judging life only from the perspective of the blindness of the human mind and understanding...then you also will be able to do the works of the Master and fulfill the thing *you* were sent to do.

It is not by what we *do* that healings occur. It is not by what we *say* that healings occur. It is not by what we pray that healings occur. *It is by what we see.*

Now this was a difficult truth for me to grasp, so entrenched was I in all I was doing, doing, doing. So why was I doing, doing, doing? All that I had done to help folks in the midst of their suffering, was it all for nothing? Was I to continue? Could, or should I continue helping them in such material ways while teaching them and reaching out with them to this new understanding? Answers to many prayers through the years continue to confirm to me that supporting folks at the conscious level of understanding that they presently hold while working with them to remove the veil that has blinded us all, is the way that has been ordained for me to go. So I have and will continue to pursue this avenue.

In the face of obvious deformity, degeneration, destruction, disease and death...behind the veil of human belief and fears...there is a fact of eternal existence that never changes. *We are His Christ.* Just as there is only One Life, there is only One Son...One manifestation of that One Life. And we are all In Him, as Him.

I am therefore under no man, no human belief or experience. Nothing has the divine authority to hold me in bondage.

As the Israelites of old, I have served and slaved under hard taskmasters, the Pharaohs of fear and disease and pain and death. But now I will serve them no more.

I have worshiped at the altar of disease, fearing its power and effect in our lives for the last time. I have served the medical madness and bowed to its authority, allowing it to do whatsoever it deemed right. But no more.

Now I *see*. And now I know.

It is truly in seeing this one Life, beyond and behind all appearances of evil, that secures to us Life and wholeness and health. This eternal Being that never changes, never can be altered and is definitely not moved by anything we have chosen to believe or fear! This is the anchor of our hope. This is the law of Life that holds us in the glory of Life Eternal now and forever.

It is this understanding which renders all disease, all evil, to be an illegitimate experience. One we have felt very vulnerable to, very victimized by, but no more!

In the same way we realize that disease is an intruder of thought, an unwanted visitor that we are not forced to entertain any longer. No more than would we allow a thief, a murder, a rapist in our home. The door is sealed; understanding and Truth stand at the door of our minds, allowing nothing but the truth to enter.

To become still enough to "feel" the eternal rhythm of all Life, is to enter in to the Present Perfection and to receive our healing.

CHAPTER TWO

THE RESURRECTION PRINCIPLE

While the earth remains, seedtime and harvest,
and cold and heat, and summer and winter, and
day and night shall not cease. If these can cease,
then my covenant of peace can fail." [1]

MANY YEARS AGO I BEGAN TO NOTICE A PATTERN, a cycle that appeared in nature. I saw it as Life always appearing after death. Or more accurately put...out of what *seems to be* death, life always appears. The understanding of this 'life principle' has brought me great comfort and assurance in my life. Thousands of healings and corrections of human discords and diseases have resulted from the unfolding and revealing of this understanding.

I watched as the seasons of winter gave way to the newness of the life of spring. Winter appeared as a death of sorts. Nothing grew... all the leaves had died and fallen off the trees. The earth energy just seemed to recede and wait. But no matter how long or how bleak the winter was, no matter how harsh and violent the time, spring always came with life and growth and the promise of goodness everywhere.

It is the same with night time. It's dark. The flowers all fold up, the birds quit singing. You can't see your nose in front of your face, except for the moon. Shadows appear everywhere, becoming whatever we image them to be.

People become afraid at night. Most of the frantic calls that I receive from my patients happen at night. Symptoms are exaggerated and exacerbated at night. It comes as a threat of death when one is already feeling alone and vulnerable. But no matter how dark and how scary the night appears, dawn always comes. The night gives way to the light without a battle or a hint of resistance. Light always overcomes darkness with no resistance. *Light is truth understood.* Once the true image of goodness and perfection and order appear, the images that darkness produced just vanish, as easily as the night gives way to the day.

But my favorite is the seed. It amazes me almost beyond words. Take for instance a black walnut seed. This is the hardest of all shells to break apart. We have two huge beautiful black walnut trees next to our house. At the end of every summer these giant seeds fall to the ground. I have even taken a hammer to these seeds and only with great force can I break one open.

Now consider this seed as representing every different seed in the earth. As it sinks deep into the ground, or is deliberately planted, image the seed becoming aware of how dark and wet and cold it is there. There is no apparent activity... and coming from the mind of the seed, no apparent way out of this darkness. "If I wiggle and squirm one way...it may not be up, and I could be wiggling down deeper instead...or sideways, and I would be wiggling forever!" How is this little seed ever going to find its way to the light of day?

Finally, in exhaustion, it ceases from all its labor and all of its fretting. *It remembers that there is a life force within it that will not rest until it has appeared.* Now, in and of itself, it is not that life force. But as sure as it exists, there is a Life energy within. To look at this seed...it is just a hard, lifeless shell, buried forever in the damp earth. But within it is the Life of eternity!

So it ceases to struggle, yields to the pulsations of the rhythm of eternal life that flows within it, and waits with great confidence. "Cast not away your confidence, which has great recompense of reward, for after you have done the will of God (which is always to surrender to that Life within) you shall receive the promise!"[2]

It took Abraham 99 years to cease his own efforts of trying to have the son born to him that God had promised. As soon as he quit struggling, trying to "make something happen," Isaac was born.

Moses spent 40 years in the wilderness of doubt and "darkness of understanding" before he finally came to the revelation of the true God at the burning bush...(that burning bush was the burning desire of his own soul to know God...that which would not be silenced until God appeared to him.) He finally needed to come to a place of trust and peaceful surrender before it could arise within his soul.

Jesus waited 30 years in the carpenter shop until he was sufficiently shed of having any confidence in himself, in his own efforts, and any trust in his own abilities, before he emerged to change the face of the entire world forever. Finally he was able to say, "I can of my own self do nothing. As I hear, that I speak, as I see, that I do."[3]

Paul spent three years in isolation after his conversion, letting go of his previously held beliefs and learning to listen to the voice of God as it revealed things that no man had ever understood before.

John spent years on the remote island of Patmos, shedding the remains of his own "selfhood" before he received the vision of the "revealing of Jesus Christ" in, to and through creation.

And King David lived in isolation tending the sheep until he learned that in every circumstance he could trust the might and power of the living God. Only then could he come forth in one day to triumph over Goliath. He later ran from Saul for years until he learned the humility and obedience to the voice of God that it would take to lead the nation as King of Israel.

So back to the little black walnut seed. When it ceases from its struggle, when it looks like there is no further life for it to live...suddenly there is a movement, a stirring from within. Divine Life is gaining momentum in strength... and from within that impossible-to-break-open seed, a crack appears in the shell. The crack gives way to a tiny sprout, with its head bent over in humility and surrender. Up, up through the heavy dirt. Up through the weight of dirt, many thousand times its own molecular weight. Up past heavy clods, rocks, and even sometimes cement that man has lain over the earth!

But this little sprout is not being motivated by its own strength. It has no strength of its own to boast. It is the strength of eternal Life that is driving it upwards, past any and every obstacle in its path. It is the same eternal Life that is *our* life and breath and purpose for existing. It knows the way and it is *relentless in its determination to be revealed to the light.*

Eventually the sprout breaks through the earth surface and continues to move upwards toward the light. Soon it lifts its head and faces the light. It opens, revealing the strength of eternal Life, coming forth as the beginning of a new walnut tree!

And Life proves, for all the world to see once again that there is no power in death. It proves that Life will not be denied its expression, in every situation and event!

It shows us the way to the resurrection of any human condition. It is in quiet surrender to the power that resides within...the presence of the eternal, unchanging wisdom of God. We are not surrendering to the condition, the disease, the evil that appears. Never!

We are surrendering to the Life that we know and believe is the *substance* of all that is created, including us. This is the resurrection principle...out of what appears to be a death of sorts...always comes life.

Once my husband and I traveled to Alaska and flew in a helicopter over the black, granite appearing mountains.

We were told that these particular mountains were formed by the lava of volcanoes centuries before. They were bleak and lifeless to me. Soon, though, we came to a stretch of land that was rich with pale green vegetation. Another mountain, but this one had recovered from the centuries of lying dormant under the weight of granite rock. Life had appeared at last!

Nothing can ever hold Life back, absolutely nothing! Its only purpose is to reveal itself in its beauty and glory...and it always does. I thought to myself as I looked out from the window of that helicopter, "Life just will not be denied!"

And I felt the presence of God smiling deep in my soul.

When I was traveling through various denominational churches in my youth, I kept hearing the phrase "death to self"...referring to the idea of self-denial. The Bible school that I attended used this doctrine to convince us that we should not want anything for our personal selves. A church I briefly visited later on used this doctrine to keep women from wearing pants, cutting their hair or wearing make-up. Many churches interpret this to mean that we are to tolerate terrible things in our lives, no matter the consequences, because it is God's will that we do so.

Let's look at what it really means.

This is why the resurrection principle is so important for us to understand. There must be a "death" to the old way of believing, the old way of seeing, the old human opinions and judgments. This is the self-denial taught to us by Jesus.

There must be a "death" to all our insane running

around frantically trying to fix our problems, or finding someone else to fix our problems. There must be a "death" to the old way of interpreting God's nature in order for any new understanding to appear.

Out from these "death" experiences, called "death to our old self initiated ideas and patterns of behavior"...the new revealing of our true nature appears. Wholeness appears, goodness appears, harmony appears, abundance appears...the Divine Life of God appears.

Remember that it is always God's purpose for His life to appear in every human situation. Always!

If there is anything within your heart that still believes that God sees you as a failure, someone who needs periods of suffering to punish, correct or direct you, you will never be able to have the confidence that is necessary to rise up out of your circumstance. You will consciously or unconsciously hold the problem to yourself.

This is what must "die" in order for Life to appear to you.

It is true that human "self" hood is a barrier to the appearing of the Divine Life. Selfishness, self-preservation, self-absorption, self-interests, etc. These capture our hearts when we are still thinking that our life is our own...that our life is our personal responsibility to figure out, that we are separate from the Life that is God...instead of a manifestation and declaration of that Life!

Darwin tells us that the first law of mankind is self-preservation. That is the first law of man seeing through the eyes of total darkness and confusion, seeing only through the human consciousness as it appears today.

But the enlightened man, who knows the mind and heart and presence and purpose of God, will never be afraid to let the self- sacrificing law of Love rule his affairs. He will never fear suffering any loss by doing so. He will know that "all things are given to him for his benefit and good," and, "all that the Father has is yours."[4] He will know that he lacks nothing...and never could... because of who he really is, and therefore never be afraid to give all that he has. The more one gives with joy and understanding...the more it flows back to him again.

There is a story in the New Testament, in the book of John, where two Greeks came to where Jesus was staying and requested to see him.[5]

Now Jesus knew that to see him as a man was really not what they were seeking...he knew that they wanted to know what made him different from anyone they had ever seen before. What Spirit motivated him? Could they ever experience the same Life that he was experiencing?

Knowing their true heart's desire, he declined to meet them in person, but said instead to one of his followers, "Go tell them that unless a kernel of wheat falls to the ground and dies, it abides alone. If it dies it will bring forth much fruit. Unless any man is willing to lose his life, he cannot gain this life that I am living. This is what the "cross" means...and it is this cross they must "take up" in order to find the Life that I am living."

Jesus was describing "death to self" or self denial...but from a high and holy view...from the vision of the Eternal Wisdom.

Once again man's literal and limited view of spiritual truths cost him great pain and confusion. Not to mention causing him to miss the glory of the Life he is intended to live here, during this very human experience.

The "little" self must die to its opinions, so that the One grand and glorious, eternal Self might appear. For we are all a reflection, a part and a manifestation of that Eternal One. That is what we must see and understand. "For as He is in heaven, so are we on the earth."[6]

Years ago I went to a lecture by a former Catholic priest. He told his story…

He had been diagnosed with liver cancer and was in the very terminal stages of that disease. He was hospitalized, and in and out of consciousness. He was wired to two IVs, one for fluids, one for blood. He had a cardiac monitor, a urinary catheter, oxygen and whatever else accompanies that scenario. His body was as yellow as a pumpkin, his eyes were sunken, his arms and legs were as skinny as a bean pole, while his abdomen was swollen and hard.

It was in this shape that he heard the Spirit of God speak to him. "Is this what you want?" When he answered, 'No," he heard,

"Then choose again."

He said in that moment he realized that God has never chosen this for man, for any reason. He realized that we are inadvertently choosing our suffering by the ideology concerning God that we hold to be true…specifically that God rewards and punishes and we have all earned punishment!

So he managed to drag himself out of bed, pulled out

his IV's, catheter, and oxygen. When the cardiac alarm went off the nurses came running, thinking they would find that he had died, but finding instead the priest trying with all his might to get his pants on. You can image the flurry he caused that day. They thought he was out of his mind because of the disease and medications. But he insisted that they let him go. The doctors were called in, the hospital administrators were called in. Finally they gave him a release form to sign and called a cab for him.

He said it was all he could do to get around his apartment, just to do the immediate care for himself. But he kept saying, "I am choosing again! I am choosing Life, no longer allowing death to rule my life. I am choosing a God of goodness and love, not a judging, punishing God. I am choosing to know that the purpose of God will be made manifest and that His Life will appear in this, as in every human circumstance."

It took 6 months of terrible struggle and "near death" times, but he finally realized strength coming back and eventually came to the end of the ordeal. Now he stood before us declaring the true nature of God and the absence of the necessity for suffering.

This is truly what the word repentance means…to chose again.

SECTION SIX

INTRODUCTION

IN SPEAKING OF TRADITIONAL RELIGION VS. the new revelation which is rising on the horizon of the human search for comprehensive understanding...

Is there a place where the old thought and the new can meet? Can this be done without losing the truths that have been established and proven? Can we hold to what is true and still embrace new understandings with a higher sense of clarity...one that will promise a life more abundant with health, with peace embracing all men, with a greater sense of purpose, with more respect to this earth we possess? Is there a place where we can see God more clearly? Where we can understand truth with a greater sense of integrity and still not lose our way? Can we honestly say that we have both understood and gained all that is available for us?

Religion has become as polarized as our politics. One side, the traditionalists, stand clinging to their established doctrines, ignoring the obvious inconsistencies, and are terrified of those who bring anything new to the table. While the other side looks back at the old with disdain, believing that they are holding their believers in bondage, wondering why people remain so blind and so afraid of seeing more. Both sides watching every word they speak, fearing lest they accidentally begin to sound like the other!

Of course, both sides are clear on issues and both sides are incomplete on issues, as is always the case when people choose an extreme position with a closed mind and an absolute disregard of the ideas of the other.

This is a time of great upheaval in religious thought. This is not of man's making although many would like to attribute it to man, thereby disregarding its importance and nullifying its significance, so that they can discount it altogether. This is God revealing a truth which has been a mystery to man since man appeared. Paul wrote of it in his book to the Ephesians, but no one understood it then either.

He called it the "mystery which has been hid in God, whereby He might gather together *all in one*, whether in heaven or in earth, all in Christ; that we might be filled with the fullness of God."[1]

As in anything new that arises from an old thought, we don't always get it right at first. We try to make the new fit into the old, because that is all we have available to relate it to. Or we become so disenchanted with the old that we don't see how it can possibly relate, so we throw out the old entirely and lose the foundation that establishes the new. That is called "throwing the baby out with the bathwater."

Another possible response when the new rises out of the old is that we enter into a kind of "cafeteria theology" where we pick and choose what we believe depending upon what we want to hear, what feels safe to us, or because some "authority" told it to us.

To those who fall into the latter category, I must quote to you these words from Isaiah: "These people do honor me with their lips, but they have removed their hearts far from me. Their understanding of me is taught by the precepts of men."[2]

I, personally, would rather listen to the struggling confusion of an honest seeker of God, than someone who simply opens their mouth and parrots whatever they have heard said.

Once we have "made up our minds" what we are going to believe and have closed our hearts to anything else, there is nothing more to say and no sense in trying. It is to *honest seekers* that we share knowledge, and together reach for understandings and new truths that will free us from our present conditions and elevate us to a "new heaven and a new earth" experience.

Once we know God as pure mercy and cease all inordinate fear of Him, once we realize that He cherishes us beyond anything we have ever felt before in our lives, we will then trust Him to lead us into greater understandings than we presently hold. We will not be afraid of where that will lead us. We will go forth with the Spirit of Truth as our guide and protector, trusting that the end of the road will be a place where God and man are *one* in thought, *one* in purpose and *one* in being.

But it is the fear of the "strange God" of punishment and wrath, judging and exacting our every move, that keeps us in bondage to the old and paralyzes us to be able to look outside of the box we have placed Him in... to really find Him. Could this be one of the "strange gods" we are warned against when we read, "Thou shall have no strange gods among you?"

Instead listen to the liberating words of God, "Behold I will send the Angel of my Presence who will go before you and lead you to the paths that I have chosen. And you shall hear a word behind you saying 'This is the way, walk you in it,' when you turn to the right hand or to the left."[3]

Now notice that you will hear a word that will lead you *when you turn this way or that*...but if you are afraid to move at all, afraid that you will stumble into something wrong, you cannot hear the word that protects and guides you. You will hear only when you trust enough to move at all.

I love what God has taught me these past many years. I love being with Divine Love and feeling so cherished and directed. I have lost my fear of God...my fear that I would be judged and condemned for anything. I walk with Love and Life now without fear and with only a sense of awe at the holiness I perceive and the hope I have gained for mankind. I no longer wait for the "other shoe to drop." There is no other shoe. I know that no hurt will ever come to me or to anyone who comes to understand God in the way that is now being revealed to us. Challenges may yet arise, but they will never cause fear or defeat. The truth has become too true for that ever to dominate us again. I have searched for the place where life can be experienced without agonies and tragedies, and this is where the search has led.

CHAPTER ONE

USHERING IN THE NEW

How does one gain such a place in consciousness, a place of fearless trust and overwhelming confidence in the goodness of God to lead and guide throughout the life-long search for unfolding truth? Is the mental understanding of the words enough? Does the constant repetition of these words finally enable us to believe them? Will that cause it to appear when we are faced with a horrible condition or situation that denies our present wholeness? Is there anything that we need to do that will contribute to this wonderful consciousness?

We find that there is nothing "to do" but much to "know."

For me, the answers are found in the life and teachings of Jesus, the Christ. Remember that the definition for the word, Christ, is the "visible expression of the invisible God." Never has there been one who more clearly demonstrated the Christ Life than Jesus. To miss his teachings is to miss the way outlined for us.

Jesus, by his words and example, clearly showed us the way to be able to easily embrace the life of perfection and glory, right here, right now. He came to reveal the true nature of God to man. He was the first to actually demonstrate that the *heart of the Lord is mercy* and not judgment. He was the one to reveal to man who we really are behind the veil of doctrine, darkness and confusion.[1] He was the first to reveal that God and man are one, and he prayed that we would come to know this, accept it and live in the glory of it.[2]

He said that "the servant is not greater than his lord, it is enough that he be *as* his lord."[3] This was a startling statement, making himself, as well as us, one with God. No wonder the religious leaders sought him to kill him!

We spoke of the old covenant and the new covenant. It was Jesus who taught us that it is by the Spirit of God alone that all these things should be manifested. He ushered in the age of Grace, saying that the nature of God would be revealed *through* us by the Spirit of God only. He brought with him a whole new way of knowing God, and a whole new way of seeing man. He proved, by the ease with which he healed, that perfect God can only bring forth perfect man. He showed us that this is the condition of our true state of being. (Remember we are human *beings*, not human *'doings'*)

He healed, to show us that God wanted us to live in freedom from the bondage and fear of disease. His healings were not to set himself above other men, but to show them what *they* are called to do and fully capable of doing. As he did, he sent them out to do likewise. He said, "As my

Father sent me, so send I you."[4] Until that time man lived under the law of right and wrong, reward and punishment, fear and guilt. It was Jesus who introduced man *into* the Law of Everlasting, perfect Life.

It was Jesus who elevated man to his rightful place as offspring of God. As the rays of the sun extend from the core sun, and contain the same light and power and brilliance as the sun itself, so are we in the glory of God.

We love and cherish Jesus for all that he taught us...for the sacrifice he lived in order for us to know the truth. It must have been difficult for him to stand alone and declare such an apparent contradiction of thought from the all pervasive religion of the elders. But so great was the Divine Love that motivated him, the sacrifice was gladly made.

He felt the heart of God as he looked out upon a world of pain and suffering and knew it was in vain. Nothing was to be gained from such an existence. There was no God who required this. Can you image the resistance he felt when declaring such truths to men, and the Love that it took to endure their resistance?

Why would men resist so great a deliverance from suffering? Why would they not openly embrace it? Why would they choose to argue for evil to be more powerful than good? Why would they not embrace a God of Love and goodness and Life? Especially when the proof was before them? Never had a man been able to do the things Jesus did to prove what he was saying was true.

These are serious questions, and the alarming truth is that *we still resist it today!*

Could it be that the Spirit of Mercy has not yet been

revealed in the hearts of those who still cling to a God of judgment, wrath and punishment?

Once when I was in Bible school, many, many years ago, I found myself caught in a place of extreme darkness. I knew I should run from the whole situation, yet felt compelled to yield to the temptation. I not only felt horrible but I lived with a sense of dread as I awaited the punishment from God that I fully expected and knew that I deserved. Instead I experienced mercy, for what I believed was the first time in my life. I remember lying on my bed one night crying, with my heart filled with condemnation and finding no place of relief, when I saw a pair of eyes looking at me with such love and mercy. I felt a tenderness that you just don't ever feel in this earth experience. Especially coming from others, who judge and condemn, thinking that they reflect the heart of God by doing so.

It was an experience that changed my way of knowing God forever. It brought with it the ability to easily walk away from the entangling situation feeling clean and innocent. This is the "goodness of God which leads men to repentance!"[5] From that time I knew that, not by punishment, but by mercy are men turned from their darkness and confusion.

Why do we confess our love for Jesus and yet deny what he told us was true about God, about us? Why do we sing praises to him and yet refuse to do the works that he said we were to do? Why are we denying the power of who we really are... and still suffer from that denial? Why are we not believing all that he spoke, and yet claim to follow him?

This is cafeteria theology. We have once again watered

down the truth. We have once again changed the truth of God to fit our present circumstances...instead of healing our present circumstances to complete the truth of God.

Truly the highest praise and thankfulness that we can demonstrate to this one who came and taught so much and sacrificed so unreservedly, is to finally accept what is true and learn to live it. And to be what we were created to be.

CHAPTER TWO

JESUS AS THE TRUTH

JESUS DECLARED THAT HE WAS THE WAY, the truth and the
Life. In this statement he was inviting us to follow him as
he explored, lived, and taught the new revelation of God...
and man in His image. It was his intention that we know
what is available for us as we walk this earth experience.
He not only taught it and lived it, he *became* the way, the
truth and the Life, so that we... *as one with him and in
him*...might enjoy the abundant life he promised us.

This concept, as being *one* with someone and actually
a part of that individual, is admittedly, difficult to grasp. It
is this concept that we must explore now, that the fullness
of these truths may become the Life we live.

The truth that Jesus demonstrated to man was that we
are all offspring of God. We come from Divinity and we are
all endowed with every attribute and characteristic of the
parent. Not after we have earned this place in God, or have
done anything to qualify for this position. Jesus taught us

that we must come to *know* God, not just about God. We must know God so that we can know ourselves.

For instance, if we see God as attacking evil with force and vengeance, we will be justified in doing the same. But if we are told that God is merciful...that is, that God sees beyond the offense of the offender and *draws from that one the goodness that is inherently there,* thereby healing the offender instead of crushing him...then we will do likewise.

So we are told not to "resist evil" but to "love your enemies." The highest expression of love is to heal the offender instead of exacting his punishment. This attitude of the heart, as taught by Jesus, is a reflection of the heart of God, thereby declaring that this is the nature of God, Himself.

We are told to pray for those who "despitefully use you and persecute you." Render good for evil. Go the second mile. Turn the other cheek. All this is so that "...you may be the offspring, the image, of your Father in Heaven, *for he sends rain on the just and unjust alike and gives of his goodness to the unthankful and the evil.*"[1] This, too, is a description of the nature of God and how God deals with His creation. By telling us this is the way we are *to live and to be* the Christ of God, He is declaring to us His nature as well.

As He does not reward and punish (but His nature is constant, not reacting to us, and is good to all) we, reflecting His image, must also not reward and punish. This sounds like condoning evil, doesn't it? It sounds like letting it exist without restraint, doesn't it?

But it isn't that at all. It is *healing the offense*...not by ignoring it, as so many are advocating these days...*but by seeing the eternal goodness that lies beyond what is seen.*

And it is hard!

It is easy to get mad, punish, retaliate and get even. It is easy to roll our eyes in judgment of another. It is easy to ignore and declare that it is "none of our business anyway!" You bet it is our business! Not to judge, not to condemn the offender, *but to heal him.* So that the true nature of that one might be released. So that Life might appear! (Robert Browning called this, "The release of the hidden Splendor!")

And so that you will have *fulfilled the reason that it came to your attention in the first place!*

Yes, that is true. Everything that comes into your experience is for you to heal it. Not to hurt you. Not to test you. Not to teach you something. (Although we always do learn from every situation) Not to judge and condemn. Not to ignore and be politically correct. *But for you to heal it.*

Jesus said, "You are the light of the world." But if that light is hid, what good is it to be a light? Unless that light shines into darkness, what purpose is there in being that light?[2]

He came and healed to show us that we have come to heal. Every man born into this world has come to heal. This is not done by judging. But this is also not done by ignoring evil when it appears. Anything that is of confusion and denies Divine Order and the eternal government of righteousness, is evil, and must be healed.

You have come to reveal what is already true and

established. "While we look not at those things which do appear, but we look at that which is hidden to appearance."[3]

Forget being politically correct. It is an excuse to be lazy and unwilling to make the sacrifice of time and Love to heal something. It is an excuse for confusion and disorder to continue to rule in the affairs of men...thereby forever concealing from them their divinity and eternal nature and oneness with all holiness and goodness.

As soon as they can receive it, we teach the patients at the clinic that they have come, not necessarily just to be healed as much as to learn to heal (which will also heal them). We tell them that this situation has come into their experience, not to hurt them, but so that the nature of God might be revealed *through them.* (Jesus allowed God to be revealed through him each time he healed, each time he spoke the words of Life.)

We allow a "one, big happy family" attitude at the clinic, not so that they can rehearse their symptoms and embellish their illness, but so that each patient will reach out to the others with compassion and deliberate healing.

Recently we had a child brought to us who was misdiagnosed with leukemia and given chemotherapy. The story was that when he was an infant and received his first immunizations, he developed a fever and had a seizure. Instead of simply bringing the fever down and thereby controlling the seizures, he was put on anticonvulsants. He must have 'fallen through the cracks' in the system because he was left on them for a long time. Soon he developed blood disorders in response to the drug and was diagnosed as being in a 'pre-leukemic' state. In the meantime he developed severe anemia and was given blood replacement. Finally, when a doctor told the family that he would need to have more chemotherapy so that "the cancer would not come back," (when he never had it in the first place) they realized that no one knew what they were doing with this child, and they left.

The child rapidly got better at the clinic and was able to run and play without pain for the first time in his little life. He smiled and talked finally, instead of cowering in the corner of the couch. But the anemia persisted.

So I asked the mother to sit with her child twice a day, in quietness and peacefulness. She was to place her hands upon him, or hold him in her arms, and just feel the love that she had for him. She was told that she had the ability to heal him and anyone who appeared within her life experience.

We all do. It is done by Love and by the intention to share the power of the Life which resides within us. We also must know the truth that each one is a manifestation of the Divine Life and therefore cannot suffer under the appearance of disorder. We were sent to do just this!

She understood and did exactly as we spoke. Within days his hemoglobin began to rise and in a few short weeks, his blood count was normal. And she was awakened to a fact of Life...of everyone's Life...that we have within each one of us the presence and power to share that Life with everyone. It will heal and we will fulfill our reason for being. We don't earn this, we don't pray for it to appear. We just *are it* and need to use it!

Another story that comes to mind happened to me many years ago while I was still a single parent raising my two daughters.

I received a letter in the mail from the IRS. It said that I had made a mistake on my tax returns and owed them an extra $700.00. Now $700.00 may not seem like much to most folks, but it may as well have been seven million to me! I tried to call them and fix it, but they wouldn't let me fix it. They just wanted me to pay or "lose my home."

I reacted in paralyzing fear, which was what they intended, of course. I stayed awake nights worrying and praying...and finally my day with the IRS agent came. I sat across a desk from a very nice lady, who turned out to be so in need of healing and love. We talked about everything from her husband's illness, to her frustrations in life, to the value of tithing. She understood what happened to my account and I was sure that she would do her best to fix it. She said to wait and see what the next letter said to do.

In the meantime I was attending a rather radical church which had really become quite militant about the evil and corruption of our government and especially the IRS. I don't remember us ever praying about this problem...just getting worked up about it. Soon they convinced me that it was my "moral duty" to fight this thing! They showed me where the IRS deliberately focuses on single parents, heads of households, to find some fault with their returns. They had me read everything available on the subject and soon I begin to attend tax-strike movements in town. Attorneys began to come out from closets to convince me that I had a "good" case against the IRS and that I should file a suit against them.

Needless to say, I got swept along with the energy of the whole mess and I sued everyone from the agent that I really liked, to the President of the United States!

The months dragged into years and I spent at least the $700.00 that I "owed" the government and probably more. The excitement was wearing off and I began to wonder what in the round world I was doing in the tax strike movement!

One day I was walking to my mailbox...I lived out in the country and it was quite a distance away. I began to pray and ask God what to do (finally). I began to realize that I was not going in the direction that He would have led me had I let Him lead at the start. I saw where I had been swept along by the "herd mentality," which was so out of my usual nature that I began to really feel disgusted with myself. While I was praying I heard, "I want you to pray for them because I love them."

I could hardly believe what I had heard. How could God love something so vile and corrupt? Wasn't *I* the one wronged here? What about justice and all?

Well, God didn't love the corruption, but he loved them. So I prayed. I had learned to see them all as despicable, so praying was hard at first. I finally broke through when I began by praying for myself...

I was wrong to listen to the advice of men. I should have asked for counsel and wisdom from the Spirit alone and waited for direction.

I was wrong to let such evil in my heart and not see beyond the wrong done to me.

I was wrong not to see the meeting that day as an opportunity to heal someone, instead of being so self absorbed.

I was wrong not to trust that Divine Love would cover and care for me in that situation.

And I was wrong to think that I needed to "take it into my own hands."

By the time I finished confessing all the ways I had "missed" the Spirit in the situation, I felt free of all the nonsense that had blocked the flow of the Spirit in the first place. Finally I was able to really pray for them.

The rest of the way to the mailbox I prayed for everyone I had met and the entire organization in general. All anger and judgment was gone, and trust and quietness had moved back into its rightful place.

I was stunned when I saw that there was a letter from the IRS in my mailbox! We had only corresponded through attorneys for so long. It said that they had decided not to pursue this situation any longer and to simply drop it. They said that I would not be hearing from them again concerning this...and I haven't.

What did I learn from all of this?

I learned that every situation was an opportunity to heal, that I would never face anything that would hurt me as long as I kept this as my focus. I learned that I was sent to heal and that was to be my only intention, no matter how the events unfolded.

I learned that I was the light...and what was the sense of being the light unless you were sent into darkness...to *be the light* that would turn the darkness into light.

I learned that it was within me to heal...because God was within me and was indeed the Life of me.

CHAPTER THREE

JESUS AS THE WAY

Not realizing the *eternal purpose* of our knowing the truth, many people now coming into this "new thought" understanding have seen it as an avenue of "getting." They seem to think that they have received these revelations of truth to bless their personal lives.

They mistakenly believe that the "abundant life" that Jesus spoke of means acquiring for themselves all that they can get. This has often become very self serving and self indulgent.

But is this the life that Jesus lived? Did he ever "use" the truth of who he was for personal gain? Is this the example of living the Christ life? Was it to "get" and accumulate as much as desired unto ones self?

There is an eternal purpose for which man was sent to this human experience and there is an eternal purpose for which the truth of his identity is revealed to him. *It is to bring the nature of God into visible expression,* that God might be revealed in and through all that is formed. It is that Divine Harmony and Infinite Order might appear throughout creation.

None of this will appear arising from such attitudes as self serving, self seeking, and self indulgence. This is "taking the name (nature) of the Lord, thy God, in vain."[1] This means using the attributes that we possess from the nature of God for our own personal gain. The word vain comes from the word "vanity." This truth was not revealed to us so that we could accumulate more and more unto ourselves, but arises from a misunderstanding of why we have come.

In healing appearances and false beliefs wherever they arise, we also heal them within ourselves. This brings certain liberty to ourselves and always causes us to experience the Life of God within us. By doing this we *do* find that the life we are living is abundant...*because it is not our life living it...*but the power and the presence of the One Eternal Life. It brings a joy and peace and sense of fulfillment with it that cannot be denied. It brings a sense of innocence and freedom from the weight of mortality beyond description.

Jesus spoke and taught for all mankind. He came to show us *how* we are to enter in to the purpose for which we have been sent and how that would bring the abundant life that he spoke of and demonstrated. He said that the way up was down, the way to win is to lose, the way to gain is to give, the first shall be last and the last first...he who seeks to save his life will surely lose it, but he who is willing to lose his life will save it.[2]

Now what is that all about?

We are talking about two identities here. There are not

really two natures, there is only one and that is God "all and in all." But we have created another nature in our minds, the nature of separation from who we are and from our oneness with our Creator and source. The Bible calls this the "sin nature." It only exists in the minds of men for it is only men who are blinded and confused on this issue. God does not enter into this confusion with us. He knows who we are!

But unfortunately man has identified himself as being a part of this sin nature. And by doing so we miss the ability to manifest who we really are and why we have come here. By doing so we also attract the suffering we believe we deserve because of our sin nature.

This is what must be lost in order to gain. We must lose this sense of life, that the true sense of Life might permeate our souls. We must 'die to this' in order to live to the new identity. This is what Paul referred to as "dying daily."[3] This is what Jesus referred to as "taking up your cross daily and following the way that I have taken." *The cross is the place where one life is exchanged for another...*or better put, one *sense* of life is given up so that the true sense of Life might be expressed.

There is no other way. "Not my will but thine be done."[4] Not by my ways and means, not by my intelligence, not by my manipulations, not by the myriads of religious exercises taught by the precepts of men, not by any way man has invented. But by a trustful, peaceful surrender to the highest expression of Christ in our lives.

Then the most wonderful thing happens, we begin to

realize that His way and our way is one and the same. We share the same wisdom, for it is all one wisdom. We share the same desires, because there is only one heart and soul and purpose.

There is a blending of mind, heart and intention...for it is the same Spirit *revealing* as the one *receiving!*

This is the way to experience life without disease or suffering. Let the mind of Wisdom live its Life. Let the Heart of Mercy freely flow. Let the Eternal purposes of the Divine Life have full expression. And you will find, as Jesus did, that there is no power in the world of form...nothing that can have dominion over you when the Eternal Life governs.

CHAPTER FOUR

THE BLOOD SACRIFICES

Recently a movie was released called, "The Passion of Christ." This caused, among other things, people to ask the question, "Why did Jesus need to go through all of that suffering? How does that free me from anything? And if it does, why are we all still suffering?"

We have heard since childhood that Jesus "died for our sins." I remember as a child sitting in church looking at a cross with Jesus hanging on it and asking Jesus why he ever allowed people to do that to him? And what did it have to do with me? How was that to have any effect upon my life?

Later as a young adult I was told that God required Jesus to die because the "justice of God needed to be fulfilled." Meaning, if someone sins, someone needs to be punished. How do I reconcile all this with my new realization that God does not reward and punish?

Further, I was told that Jesus willingly died in my behalf, so that I wouldn't be punished for my sins. Right from the start that confused me. If that was true, why were we all still suffering and dying? Was there something more that needed to be done? Something that I was supposed to do? I was told by some that Jesus did it all and there was nothing that I needed to do. Others told me that I needed to "walk worthy of the sacrifice," meaning to live as "good" as I possibly could.

Another source of confusion came at a much later date. When God began to teach me about who I really was, that I was actually created in His image and that He only acknowledged that as my true identity…if God in mercy, only sees me as He created me, and "does not attribute sin to my account," why, then, was the sacrifice necessary?

To really do these questions justice, we must travel back in time when the method of approaching God was through a blood sacrifice. The more fervent was the desire to "reach" God, the greater number of animals were sacrificed.

To begin we must understand the phrase, "The life is in the blood."[1] This means that the *nature of any species, including man, is considered "in the blood."*

The Old Testament Israelites were told not to consume the blood of any animal. In other words, they were not to partake of the "nature" of any animal. Looking at the spiritual significance of this we must understand that each animal possessed a specific nature, which corresponded with the nature of the "natural man."

For instance, the bull was symbolic of the stubborn, self willed aspect of the natural man. So when the bull was sacrificed, it depicted man sacrificing his self will in order to gain access to God. So the "offering of the bull" in sacrifice to God was always required every morning and before every prayer, every event, every single time man needed to communicate with God. This is called the Burnt offering. The Burnt offering was significant in that it was the only sacrifice where the entire animal was to be reduced to ashes.[2]

Spiritually speaking this is very important to us in that we also must surrender the entirety of our human will in order to realize the presence of God, although God is always present. It is the single most important step to hearing the voice of God, or "realizing the impulse of Spirit." Without this step our will collides with the will of God and we cannot discern Divine direction, wisdom or counsel.

Now here is the question that separates the old religious doctrines from the new understanding. This is the Achilles tendon of religion, so to speak.

Who really needed this sacrifice?

God or man? If God declared that it was necessary, as we are so often told, was it to appease his justice and anger at man? Or were they given this ritual in order to enable them to communicate with God, by symbolically removing the strong, stubborn will of the "natural" man?

We find that these sacrifices were for the benefit of man, and not to appease an angry God, as we have been led to believe.

Nor because God required that "something must die for our sins."

Another animal sacrificed was the goat. The most significant thing I know about a goat is that it will eat anything! Once when I visited a goat farm to pick up goat milk for a patient of mine, I ducked into the barn to look at some baby goats. When I returned to my car in about 20 minutes, the goats had eaten the chrome bumper off the front of my car!

When we listen to the doctrines and ideas of man, whatever is blowing in the wind at any given time, and we do not ask counsel from God alone, we are "eating" what ever is out there. Usually we would rather "eat" whatever others are eating, than to take the time and effort and dedication to truth that it takes to ask for Divine Wisdom in any matter, and wait until it appears to us. It's easier, but mostly wrong.

King David often said that he "would rather sit alone in the house of God (Divine Consciousness) than to sit at the banquet table with fools." And this is what he meant.

Another thing I found out about goats was while I was still in Bible school. We lived on an eighty five acre farm and one of my jobs at the farm was to care for the goats. Every Saturday morning I would walk with my girls over to the area where the animals were kept and we would bathe the goats, trim their hoofs, and in general take care of whatever their needs were.

One day I could hear the goats crying and bleating from a mile away. When I arrived at the barn area I could see that one of the goats had her head caught in some chicken wire that had entangled itself around the fence. The other goats were backing off and then charging her, ramming her sides. She was pouring blood and wailing. I ran as fast as I could and rescued her, driving the rest of the herd away. We spent hours patching her up.

When I finished I asked the guys who worked the farm area why that happened? They told me that animals destroyed their own when trapped or wounded, weak or frail. Only the strong survived to carry on the species. Man! I thought, "If I felt that way, Lara (my youngest daughter) would not be here today!"

But then I realized how we also destroy our weak and fragile. Every time we judge someone who is acting out from their distorted image of themselves; every time we talk about offenses or weakness of another; and every time we withhold forgiveness, retaliate or react to another's attack, giving energy to the very thing which is destroying them.

Remember we are sent to heal, never to agree with error when it appears. Every time we agree with someone who believes that they are weak, sick, poor, lost, etc., we are encouraging their destruction...not healing them by seeing beyond appearances to their true and unchangeable nature.

When we cease to do these things, we are sacrificing the "goat" nature. Also when we cease to follow the crowd, but learn to walk with Love and Truth, seeking Wisdom and Counsel from Spirit only, we are sacrificing the "goat" nature.

Turtledoves, another common animal sacrificed, represent Love. They mate for life. They represent devotion and commitment. When they were sacrificed, the offering was a dedication to fulfillment of Divine purpose, no matter what.

You are probably getting it already, but let's do one more.

❧

What do we know about sheep? They are considered to represent the nature of Christ more than any other animal. They are obedient in that they will follow their shepherd wherever he takes them. They are non-combative. They possess no defense mechanism for self protection. They are so focused upon their shepherd, that they do not see a need for defense. They are the picture of innocence, submission and gentleness. When we choose this thought as the truth of our lives, we are offering this to the *purpose of God* in the earth. This is our Lamb sacrifice. This is why Jesus is referred to as the Lamb of God.

Years later, *Jesus lived and became all of these sacrifices.* He did it to show us that this was the way we were to follow. *This was the heart of the whole message.* We were to offer the old image of man, deny its power and substance, and refuse to be influenced by it any longer. Refuse to bow to its power over us. This is the cross...the place where one life is exchanged for another. We were to do this daily...offer the old so that the new might appear.

We do this every time we choose to heal instead of judge. We do this every time we make a choice to see past the visible to the heart of the invisible.

We do this every time we yield our will and way to follow the wisdom of God. We do this every time we refuse to follow the herd mentality of world thought and choose to wait for Divine direction.

We do this every time we are confronted with evil and do

not "lift up our sword" to react, but pause to heal the situation instead.

❧

This is the significance of the "sacrifices" for us now. This is how they are fulfilled in each life. This is a far cry from the current religious doctrines that declare that God's justice required that something "die for the sins of mankind!" If "sin" means having a "sense of separation from our true identity," then dying to this thought, or nature, will in fact be the fulfillment of "dying for the sins."

Jesus fulfilled these sacrifices daily and we are to do the same, **for we are all part of the One Life that he lived.** His "cross" was carried daily and hourly. The final cross experience was proof that when we allow this Divine Life to appear, when we commit ourselves to this end, even death cannot hold us! This is the power that overcomes even death.

Although religious doctrines have for centuries declared that it was God who required this sacrifice for the sins of the world, we can readily see that it was *we* who needed this and not God. It was we who needed to let go of one image of man so that the true image might appear.

As we mentioned in an earlier chapter, right in the middle of the era of animal sacrifices, King David declared, "Sacrifice and offering for sins you do not require. But my ears have you opened."[3] Again realizing that a life of relationship and communication, a life of trust and confidence in the purposes of God, was all that was really necessary.

Later Paul said, "Sacrifices and offerings for sin you do not require, but a body have you prepared for me. Lo, I have come to do your will, Oh God."[4] In this Paul was saying that an understanding of the One Life manifested (Jesus) as One body, (spiritual body of Christ...us) which has surrendered to the mind and purpose of God, is all that is needed for fulfillment.

This settles the question of who would benefit from the sacrifice...who it was that needed a "death of one consciousness that a more pure consciousness could arise."[5]

CHAPTER FIVE

JESUS AS THE LIFE

JUST AS THERE IS ONLY ONE ETERNAL, pure and perfect Life, there is only one representation of that life on earth... and that is called the "SON." This is also referred to as the Christ.

We refer to Jesus as the "only begotten Son," yet we know now that we also are the Christ of God, or the sons of God. How is this apparent confusion reconciled? By knowing this...we are *in Him, in Jesus*, as the Christ...the visible expression of the one life.[1]

That means that since there is only one son, we all are a part of that one son. We are now, and have always been, that one son. It is a "many membered son."[2]

Just as you have one body, but that body has many varied parts, all completing your one body...so also is Christ.

God is all in all. One life seen and expressed as one son.

When Jesus willingly sacrificed the conscious image of the sin nature...*the whole consciousness of sin was erased from us all.* How? **Because we are all in him...one son, one Christ.**

What I am about to say is difficult to grasp unless you realize that eternity does not embrace time. Time is something we invented to give us orientation to our human existence. Time does not exist in eternity.

Taking this understanding of one life, one son, to its fullness of expression...

We were in him when he was born in the stable.

We were in him when he grew up in the carpenter shop.

We were in him when he was baptized at the Jordon River. ("Buried with him in baptism... wherein you were also raised with him.")[3]

We were in him when he taught, when he healed, when he prayed.

We were in him at the palace of Pilate.

We were in him every time he gave up the human will to fulfill the Divine purpose of God.

We were in him at the last supper, garden of Gethsemane, and at the hill of Calvary.

We were in him when he, once and for all...*as us all*...gave up every last remnant of the human consciousness to take on the Eternal Mind of God.

And most important for us to know, we were in him when he rose from the dead, declaring that nothing of death, no sin, no sickness, no darkness at all, could ever have dominion over us again.

That is why we call him Savior.

That is why we can say, we now posses the mind of God,

the Spirit of Truth and we walk as the Christ of God...the visible expression of the invisible God. This is why we read, "we are *now* seated at the right hand of God (power)...all of the seeming power of earth is *now* under our feet."[4]

That is why we can declare ourselves one with the Father, as the *one son* in the earth.[5]

This is why no evil can empower us.

This is why no sickness can hold us.

This is why we can live above the doctrines of sin and suffering.

This is why nothing of this earth can dominate us... or in any way empower us... to enslave us ever.

It is done. It is truly finished.

REFERENCES

INTRODUCTION
[1]Genesis 3:10–11, *24*

SECTION 1

CHAPTER 1
[1] Matthew 9:17, *29*

CHAPTER 2
[1] Hosea 6:6, *34*
[2] Jeremiah 9:24, *34*
[3] Matthew 5:8, *36*
[4] Titus 1:15, *36*
[5] II Samuel 22:26, *36*

CHAPTER 3
[1] Genesis 1:31, *38*
[2] Genesis 1:11,12, *38*
[3] Psalms 100:3, *38*
[4] Luke 17:21, *41*
[5] Isaiah 11:9, *41*
[6] Romans 8:19–22, *41*
[7] Isaiah 11:6–8, *41*
[8] Isaiah 65:17–25, *41*
[9] II Timothy 2:13, *41*

CHAPTER 4
[1] Matthew 9:29, *42*

CHAPTER 5
[1] Psalms 100:3, *45*
[2] Genesis 1:27, *45*
[3] Deuteronomy 30:20, *45*
[4] Isaiah 43:7, *46*
[5] I Corinthians 6;19, *47*
[6] Job 1:1, *47*
[7] Job 42:5, *49*
[8] Psalms 139:14, *50*

CHAPTER 6
[1] John 9:39–41, *53*

CHAPTER 7
[1] John 13:3–10, *54*

CHAPTER 10
[1] Luke 6:6, *70*
[2] Ecclesiastes 3:14, *72*
[3] Proverbs 23:7, *73*
[4] I Corinthians 2;16, *75*
[5] Genesis 30:31–43, *76*
[6] Genesis 33:10, *77*

To learn more about Michele O'Donnell's work and "Living Beyond Disease" check out our website www.micheleodonnell.com.

To order other "Living Beyond Disease" products or to be placed on our mailing list please contact us at the number below or fill out the form and mail it to:

LA VIDA PRESS
1815 San Pedro Avenue • San Antonio, TX 78212 • 888-493-8660

Of Monkeys and Dragons: Freedom from the Tyranny of Disease
(Book #1 in LBD trilogy)

		QUANTITY	SUBTOTAL
Soft Back—English	$12.95	____	____
Soft Back—Spanish	$12.95	____	____
Hard Back—English	$21.95	____	____
Audio book—6 CD's	$29.95	____	____

The God That We've Created: The Basic Cause of All Disease
(Book #2 in LBD trilogy)

Soft Back—English	$12.95	____	____
Hard Back—English	$21.95	____	____

"Living Beyond Disease" audio cassette teaching series
Cassette Teaching Tapes (See website or call for list. Over 100 available)

Albums (10 tapes)	$60.00	____	____
Single Tapes	$ 6.00	____	____

"Living Beyond Disease" video teaching series

6–30 minute DVD's	TBA	____	____

SUBTOTAL ____

SHIPPING/HANDLING $3.95 PER ITEM ____
(Call for single tape S&H)

TOTAL ____

Name: _____

Address: _____

_____

Phone: _____ Email: _____

Check # _____ or Credit Card: _____ exp. date _____

Signature: _____

____ Please add me to the "Living Beyond Disease" mailing list
____ Please send me information on the next "Living Beyond Disease" annual retreat
____ Please send me information about the quarterly "Living Beyond Disease" newsletter

To learn more about Michele O'Donnell's work and "Living Beyond Disease" check out our website www.micheleodonnell.com.

To order other "Living Beyond Disease" products or to be placed on our mailing list please contact us at the number below or fill out the form and mail it to:

LA VIDA PRESS
1815 San Pedro Avenue • San Antonio, TX 78212 • 888-493-8660

Of Monkeys and Dragons: Freedom from the Tyranny of Disease
(Book #1 in LBD trilogy)

		QUANTITY	SUBTOTAL
Soft Back—English	$12.95	_____	_____
Soft Back—Spanish	$12.95	_____	_____
Hard Back—English	$21.95	_____	_____
Audio book—6 CD's	$29.95	_____	_____

The God That We've Created: The Basic Cause of All Disease
(Book #2 in LBD trilogy)

Soft Back—English	$12.95	_____	_____
Hard Back—English	$21.95	_____	_____

"Living Beyond Disease" audio cassette teaching series
Cassette Teaching Tapes (See website or call for list. Over 100 available)

Albums (10 tapes)	$60.00	_____	_____
Single Tapes	$ 6.00	_____	_____

"Living Beyond Disease" video teaching series

6–30 minute DVD's	TBA	_____	_____

SUBTOTAL		_____
SHIPPING/HANDLING $3.95 PER ITEM		_____
(Call for single tape S&H)		
TOTAL		_____

Name: _____

Address: _____

_____

Phone: _____ Email: _____

Check # _____ or Credit Card: _____ exp. date _____

Signature: _____

___ **Please add me to the "Living Beyond Disease" mailing list**
___ **Please send me information on the next "Living Beyond Disease" annual retreat**
___ **Please send me information about the quarterly "Living Beyond Disease" newsletter**